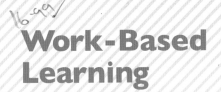

Work-Based Learning

16-99

HAIRDRESSING & BEAUTY THERAPY

Christine McMillan-Bodell

Samantha Taylor

ALWAYS LEARNING

PEARSON

Heinemann is an imprint of Pearson Education Limited, Edinburgh Gate, Harlow, Essex, CM20 2JE.

www.pearsonschoolsandfecolleges.co.uk

Heinemann is a registered trademark of Pearson Education Limited

Text © Christine McMillan-Bodell and Samantha Taylor

Designed by Dickidot Limited/ am designs

Typeset by Kamae Design

Original illustrations © Pearson Education 2011

Illustrated by Artful Doodlers and Mark Watkinson

Cover design by Wooden Ark

Cover image: Getty images: Larysa Dodz

Printed and bound in Spain by Graficas Estella

Index by Indexing Specialists (UK) Ltd.

The rights of Christine McMillan-Bodell and Samantha Taylor to be identified as authors of this work have been asserted by them in accordance with the Copyright, Designs and Patents Act 1988.

First published 2011

15 14 13 12 11

10 9 8 7 6 5 4 3 2 1

British Library Cataloguing in Publication Data

A catalogue record for this book is available from the British Library

ISBN 978 0 435 07488 3

Websites

There are links to relevant websites in this book. In order to ensure that the links are up-to-date, that the links work, and that the sites aren't inadvertently linked to sites that could be considered offensive, we have made the links available on our website at www.pearsonhotlinks.co.uk. Search for the title Level 1 NVQ Diploma Hairdressing and Beauty Therapy or ISBN 9780435074883.

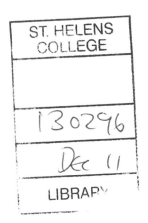

Contents

Acknowledgements

The publisher would like to thank the following for their kind permission to reproduce their photographs:

(Key: b-bottom; c-centre; l-left; r-right; t-top)

Alamy Images: Kim Karpeles 74, Shopics 76; **Carlton Professional:** Carlton Professional 27r, 253; **Getty Images:** Giulio Marcocchi 186b, Gregor Schuster Photographers Choice 217; **Pearson Education Ltd:** Ann Veck 196/1, Denman 139c, Gareth Boden 18, 27l, 111, 130, 139l, 139r, 157, Hairtools 139t, image source 34, 122, 148, 162, Image source 134, Jules Selmes 153t, 261cl, Mind Studio 19l, 19cl, 19cr, 19r, 30, 47, 50, 85/3, 101l, 101c, 101r, 118, 144tl, 144tc, 144tr, 144bl, 144bc, 144br, 145tl, 145tc, 145tr, 145bl, 145bc, 145br, 176l, 176r, 179, 182/1, 182/2, 182/3, 182/4, 183/5, 183/6, 185/1, 185/2, 185/4, 186/1, 186/2, 186/3, 186/4, 186/5, 186/6, 186/7, 192t, 192b, 193, 194, 196/2, 196/3, 196/4, 196/5, 196/6, 220, 224, 306/1, 306/2, 306/3, 306/4, 307/5, 307/6, 307/7, 307/8, 308/9, 308/10, 308/11, 308/12, 309/13, 309/14, 309/15, 309/16, 312/1, 312/2, 312/3, 312/4, 313/5, 313/6, 313/7, 313/8, 314/9, 314/10, 314/11, 314/12, 315/13, 315/14, 315/15, 315/16, Stuart Cox 36, 65, 75, 86, 110, 133, 219, 238/1, 238/2, 238/3, 238/4, 239/5, 239/6, 239/7, 239/8, 240/9, 240/10, 240/11, 240/12, 241/13, 241/14, 241/15, 241/16, 242/17, 242/18, 242/19, 242/20, 243/21, 243/22, 243/23, 243/24, , 244/25, 244/26, 244/27, 244/28, 255, 272/1, 272/2, , 272/3, 272/4, 273/5, 273/6, 273/7, 273/8, 274/10, 274/11, 274/12, 274t/12, 289l, 289r, Studio 8. Clark Wiseman 205r, Stuart Cox 274/9, Tony & Guy 102, Tudor photography 109, 170, 112, 114/1, 114/2, 115/3, 115/4, 116/2, 116/3, 117/1, 117/2, 119/1, 119/2, 119/3, 119/4, 120/5, 120/6, 120/7, 125, 153b, 154, 159, 167, 171t, 171b; **Science Photo Library Ltd:** Dr M A Ansary 293br, Dr P Marazzi 230bl, 230br, 231tl, 231br, 292bl, 293tl, 293tr, 293bl, Dr P. Marazzi 230tl, Ian Hooton 231tr, Jane Shemit 231bl, 292br, Science Photo Library 106, 107, 292tl, 292tr, St Bartholomew's Hospital 230tr; **Shutterstock.com:** Alena Ozerova 250, Apollofoto 261l, Darren Hubley 209, Dasha Petrenko 174, dpaint 188, Jason Stitt 72, 205l, Junial Enterprises 320, Marc Dietrich 278, Monkey Business Images 261cr, Payless Images 56, Rade Kovac 33, Valua Vitaly 266, Vibrant Image Studio 198, Yuri Arcurs 8, 203, 214

Cover images: *Front:* **Getty Images:** Larysa Dodz

All other images © Pearson Education

Every effort has been made to trace the copyright holders and we apologise in advance for any unintentional omissions. We would be pleased to insert the appropriate acknowledgement in any subsequent edition of this publication.

Introduction

Why choose a career in hairdressing and beauty therapy?

Hairdressing and beauty therapy offer opportunities and choice throughout your working life. Once you have qualified and gained your skills you can take them wherever you want, whenever you want. If you are thinking about a career in hairdressing, an exciting future in a high-tech industry may be waiting for you, with the chance to become your own boss or to work in another role such as image consultant, sales representative, wig-maker, salon manager, colour technician or perm technician. If you are thinking about a career in beauty therapy, you could be using your skills while cruising the world on a luxury liner, working as a make-up artist, or running your own beauty salon business. The opportunities in the beauty industry are amazing, but you must be prepared to work hard and show dedication to the industry. If you are ready to do this, you will have the opportunity for new and exciting experiences.

 Salon life

Jasmina completed her Level 1 (NVQ) Certificate in Beauty Therapy before moving on to complete Levels 2 and 3. She is now working on a cruise liner carrying out beauty and complementary therapies on the passengers. Her days are very long but very rewarding. Jasmina has decided that her next career move should be trying for a job as an airline therapist as she has got the travel bug and fancies travelling around the world while working in a job she loves.

How to use this book

Level 1 NVQ Diploma Hairdressing and Beauty Therapy will introduce you to the basics of hairdressing and beauty therapy. It covers all the relevant performance criteria and range statements linked to the latest National Occupational Standards required to complete the Level 1 Diploma in Hairdressing and Beauty Therapy.

It includes the latest units in blow-drying, plaits and twists and hair colouring as well as skin treatments, make-up and nail services. Illustrated step-by-step instructions will help you learn a variety of practical procedures while introductory units cover what you will need to know about working in a salon. You will also learn about the science of hair as well as essential information on anatomy and physiology that will underpin the skills you are learning at Level 1.

The book is divided into three sections:

In the Workplace contains all the units which relate to your work with clients and colleagues, as well as your responsibilities in the salon.

Practical Skills Hair will help you gain the skills which are essential for hairdressing.

Practical Skills Beauty provides guidance on how to carry out treatments.

To help you achieve each unit of work, the book contains:

- *Get up and go!* features to involve you in an active role in your learning and development
- *Salon life* features to help you think about the practicalities of hairdressing and beauty therapy and the type of situations you will have to deal with every day
- *Memory jogger* features to test your knowledge so you know what you might need to brush up on

- *Get ahead* features to help you make the step from Level 1 through to Level 2, preparing you for the world of work which lies ahead
- *Top tips* features giving you helpful information about good practice.

What is an NVQ/SVQ?

A National Vocational Qualification (NVQ) or a Scottish Vocational Qualification (SVQ) is made up of separate units that set out exactly what you must be able to do, and to what standard.

The practical work you carry out will be linked to the performance criteria in each unit, and the assessor will mark you against the standards set by the awarding body. This means you must carry out certain practical activities to the standard set out by the awarding body, and your assessor will help you with this.

Each unit is worth a certain amount of credit. To gain a Level 1 Diploma in Hairdressing and Beauty Therapy you **must** achieve **five** mandatory units totalling 17 credits and optional units that add up to a minimum of 24 credits.

Mandatory Units

G20 Make sure your own actions reduce risks to health and safety (4 credits)

G3 Contribute to the development of effective working relationships (4 credits)

B1 Prepare and maintain salon treatment work areas (3 credits)

GH1 Shampoo and condition hair (4 credits)

GH3 Prepare for hair services and maintain work areas (2 credits)

Optional Units

G2 Assist with salon reception duties (4 credits)

GH2 Blow-dry hair (4 credits)

GH4 Assist with hair colouring services (4 credits)

GH5 Assist with perming hair services (3 credits)

GH6 Plait and twist hair using basic techniques (4 credits)

GH7 Remove hair extensions (3 credits)

B2 Assist with facial skin care treatments (4 credits)

B3 Assist with day make-up (4 credits)

N1 Assist with nail services (4 credits)

NVQ/SVQ structure

All NVQs/SVQs have the same structure, which includes:

- **Units.** These are the subjects that you will be learning about. For example, when learning about reception skills for Level 1, the unit is called: Unit G2 Assist with salon reception duties.

- **Elements.** Each unit is made up of elements. For example, Unit G2 Assist with salon reception duties is made up of: Maintain the reception area; Attend to clients and enquiries; Help to make appointments for salon services.

- **Performance criteria.** These describe the activities, either theory or practical, that you need to carry out in order to complete the unit successfully.

- **Range statements.** These are the situations that must be covered in your learning, for example, the type of client, type of treatment or booking method (phone or face-to-face).

- **Knowledge and understanding.** This is the background knowledge that you must know so that you can carry out the treatment or activity competently.

- **Evidence.** Evidence is proof of your learning. It can be coursework, assignments, client letters, drawings, photos or tutor comments. Most evidence will be signed by your assessor, to confirm that it is correct and your own work.

These need to be gathered in a portfolio as proof of your learning and progress.

Assessment – How you will be assessed

Practical: For each unit that you practise your skills in you will need to be assessed. Usually this will be through observation of your practical skills by your assessor, and if you prove that you are safe and competent you will pass the assessments.

Theory: You will also need to keep a portfolio of evidence; this will be a file containing information to show that you have covered all of the necessary knowledge requirements to be able to carry out your practical skills. This will be recorded in a candidate handbook which will be signed by an assessor.

As well as your practical assessments and portfolio of evidence you will need to do assignments and sit tests on various units for your qualification.

 Top tips

Points to think about when putting your portfolio together:

1 Does it have an attractive front cover, e.g. magazine cuttings, clear bold writing, and lots of colour and design?

2 Does it have an organised, easy-to-understand contents page and clear page numbers throughout?

3 Does it contain clear and neat notes from each lesson, either handwritten or word-processed?

4 Does it include interesting articles on health and beauty subjects?

5 Does it contain a conclusion – your comments at the end of the portfolio on:
- what you learned or gained from the course
- how much you enjoyed the course
- whether you are intending to progress further to Level 2
- any other information you think might be useful?

UNIT G20

Make sure your own actions reduce risks to health and safety

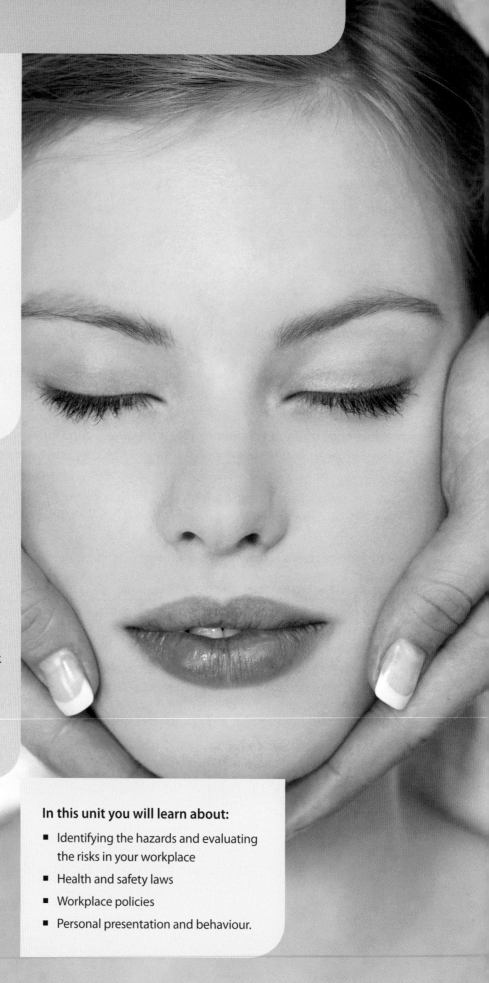

Hairdressing and Beauty therapy is an exciting, fast-moving industry, but just as it presents you with some great opportunities, it also involves responsibilities. You will be working with clients and using certain tools and products, and there are procedures that you must follow in order to ensure that your actions do not create any health and safety hazards and that you do not ignore hazards that present risks in your workplace.

Your health and safety responsibilities at work include making sure that your actions protect the health and safety of yourself and others, meet any legal responsibilities and follow workplace instructions.

In this unit you will learn about:

- Identifying the hazards and evaluating the risks in your workplace
- Health and safety laws
- Workplace policies
- Personal presentation and behaviour.

Here are some key terms you may meet in this unit:

Hazard –
something with the
potential to cause harm

Risk –
the likelihood that a hazard
will actually cause harm

Control –
how risks are identified,
managed and then reduced
to acceptable levels

Legislation –
a law or laws passed
by an official body

Negligence –
carelessness and
lack of attention

Fire risk assessment –
a formal check to identify what
the dangers of fire are and what
can be done to prevent a fire

Assembly point –
an agreed meeting place
outside a building

Premises –
a place of business

**Health and Safety Executive
(HSE) –**
the government body that is
in charge of making the rules
governing health and safety

Disinfection –
use of a chemical that
cuts down bacteria and
micro-organisms

Sterilisation –
a procedure that kills
micro-organisms

Evacuate –
leave an area or premises
in an orderly fashion

Flammable –
something that can
very easily catch fire

Precautions –
things you can do in
advance to stop
something happening

Cross-infection –
when germs or bacteria
are transferred from one
person to another

Identifying the hazards and evaluating the risks in your workplace

This unit covers the health and safety responsibilities for everyone in the hair and beauty therapy industry. You have to be aware of specific **legislation** for your particular job role. The Health and Safety at Work Act (HASWA) 1974 (see page 12 for more information) covers everyone in the salon, and it is important that you know and understand your responsibilities under this act. You must always make sure that your actions do not create a health and safety risk. In the workplace, many things can cause accidents, injury or illness if they are not recognised and made safe.

Risk assessment and control

Risk assessment and control are the responsibility of everyone and any health and safety risks you spot should be reported immediately. For your own safety, you cannot always act upon the risk, and in such cases you will have to inform a higher authority so that it can be dealt with.

It is crucial that you understand the terms '**hazard**', '**risk**' and '**control**'.

- A hazard is something with the potential to cause harm; something that could cause an accident or injury.

- A risk is the likelihood that the hazard will actually cause harm; the threat of something dangerous happening because of the hazard.

- Control refers to the measures that you put into place to remove risks or to reduce them to acceptable levels.

Almost anything may be a hazard, but may or may not become a risk. Some hazards could be thought of as 'accidents waiting to happen', as they pose such a high risk. Other hazards are less of a risk, but need to be identified and controlled nevertheless.

For example, in a salon, many deliveries are made. If some boxes of products were delivered and set down on the floor beside reception, these boxes would be a hazard. The risk would be the chance that someone could trip over the boxes and hurt themselves. The risk would be high if the boxes were in the middle of the floor, directly in the path of the staff and clients in the salon, but the risk could be controlled by moving the boxes to a place where they are less likely to be in the way of people who are moving about in the salon.

You need to be aware of the hazards that may exist in your workplace, and you will need to be able to spot hazards, identify the risks that they pose, and take steps to make sure that they do not cause a problem to you, your clients or other staff.

>> **Get up and go!**

On page 11 is a table giving you examples of hazards which present risks. Read the table of hazards and risks and, for each situation, complete the table by stating how you would make it safer and less likely to turn into an accident or injury, i.e. how you would control the risk.

Hazard	Risk	Control measure
Electrical leads trailing on the floor	Tripping over leads	Run flexes alongside the wall
A light bulb that has blown	Accidents because of poor light	
Highly polished floors	Slipping	
Badly fitting carpet or lino	Tripping up	
Trolleys and desks overloaded with equipment and products	Furniture tipping over	
Plugs that have loose or frayed leads	Possible electric shock or risk of fire	
Rushing about too much, without concentrating	Bumping into people and causing an injury	
Staff carrying tools in the pocket of her uniform	Cuts or wounds if someone bumps into her	
Carrying too much at once	Can't see where you are going which results in an accident or a bad back	
Breakages or spills that are not cleared up instantly	Cuts or slipping over	
Unsterilised tools	**Cross-infection**	

Remember that you will not be able to deal with all **hazards** yourself. Work within the limits of your own authority and if you are unable to deal with a problem, report it and be clear and concise in your information to the person who is responsible. Do not ignore it, hoping it will go away, as you may endanger another person.

? Memory jogger

1 Who is responsible for health and safety in the workplace?

2 What do the letters HASWA stand for?

3 What is a risk and what is a hazard? Give two examples of each.

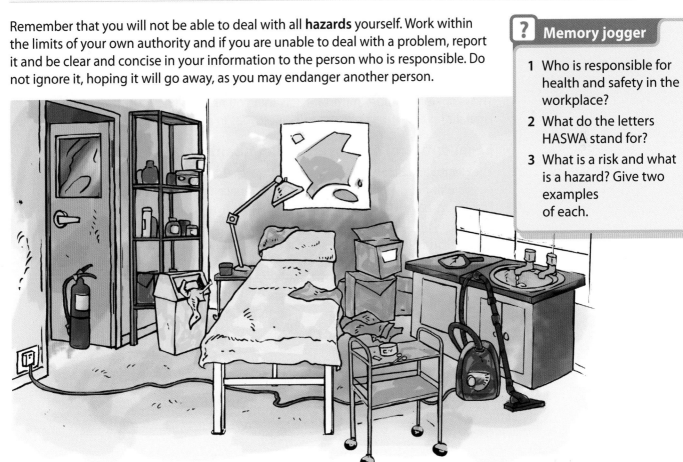

How good are you at spotting a hazard? Identify the hazards in the salon shown and make a list of them. How many did you spot?

Health and safety laws (1)

Every workplace, whether it is a shop, office, factory or beauty salon, must follow a set of health and safety rules laid down by the **Health and Safety Executive (HSE)**. These rules are designed to protect employers, employees and clients from accident, illness and injury. The most relevant acts for hairdressing and beauty therapy are listed below.

- The Health and Safety at Work Act 1974 (HASWA).
- The Fire Precautions (WorkPlace) Regulations 1997.
- The Electricity at Work Regulations 1989.
- The Gas Safety (Installation and Use) Regulations 1998.
- The Manual Handling Operations Regulations 1992.
- The Personal Protective Equipment at Work Regulations 1992.
- The Control of Substances Hazardous to Health Regulations 2002 (COSHH).
- The Health and Safety (First Aid) Regulations 1981.
- The Environmental Protection Act 1990, Waste Regulations 1992 and Special Waste Regulations 1996.
- The Reporting of Injuries, Diseases and Dangerous Occurrences Regulations 1995 (RIDDOR).
- The Local Government (Miscellaneous Provisions) Act 1982.

The Health and Safety at Work Act 1974 (HASWA)

This is one of the most important acts that you need to know about. It covers the legal duties of both employers and employees in all workplaces.

Legal duties of employers under health and safety law

The Health and Safety at Work Act 1974 states that an employer must do everything possible to provide a safe and healthy workplace with adequate welfare facilities. Employers have a legal duty to make sure that everyone is kept healthy, safe and well at work. It is a legal duty to follow these and if a business is found negligent it can be prosecuted.

Legal duties of employees under health and safety law

The **HSE** (Health and Safety Executive, the government body that makes the rules regarding health and safety) also expects all employees to play their part in taking reasonable care of their own and others' health and safety. Your responsibilities are outlined in the Health and Safety Law poster. Failure to follow the act can result in serious consequences and you should be aware that heavy fines and/or imprisonment can result if the act is ignored. If you have any worries about healthy and safety, talk them through with someone more senior. Make sure that your concerns are recorded, and any action required is followed up.

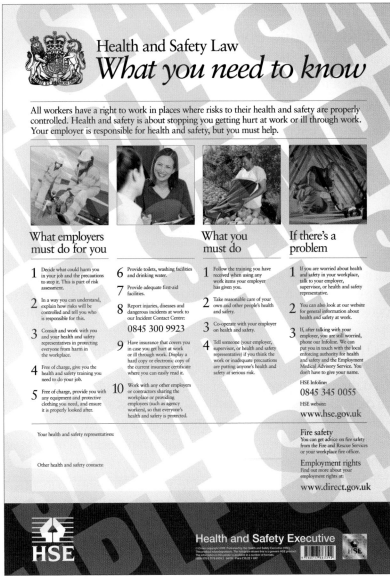

The Health and Safety Law poster (Source: Health and Safety Executive)

Top tip

For further information visit the Health and Safety Executive website. You can access this by going to www.pearsonhotlinks.co.uk and searching for this title.

Get ahead

Search the Internet to see if you can find any beauty therapy businesses that have been fined or prosecuted because they have not followed the Health and Safety at Work Act. The businesses could include salons, spas, product retailers, product manufacturers and so on.

Health and safety laws (2)

Hot and cold running water

The salon must have a constant supply of hot and cold running water. For Beauty Therapy treatment rooms should have a separate sink with hot and cold running water. However, if a large treatment room has been separated into treatment bays by curtains, then a central sink will do.

The water supply is used for sanitising hands and tools, cleaning the salon, and for parts of the treatment, for example, mask removal or shampooing hair.

Your responsibilities at work: working with water

Report to your supervisor *immediately*:

- blocked sinks, so that they don't overflow
- water that comes out of the tap an unusual colour
- any leak, loose tap or cracked pipe.

Don't:

- leave taps running, especially the hot water tap as this is wasteful and very expensive for the salon
- flush mask products or other semi-solid products down the sink

> **Top tip** ✓
>
> Dirty water smells unpleasant and encourages the growth of bacteria, which can cause illness.

Staff areas

Your employer has a duty to provide a space in which employees can rest and eat. A staff room or separate area is important because it is not acceptable to eat in the reception or client areas. Even drinks in the salon should be reserved for clients, in order to maintain a professional image.

The staff room should have an area for staff coats and preferably lockers for valuables such as handbags and expensive tools. A separate toilet and washing facility would also be ideal, but this is not always possible and staff may have to share the toilet with clients. If this is the case, staff must give their clients preference and make sure that they leave the room spotless at all times.

A staff area with comfortable seating, tea- and coffee-making facilities and a microwave would also benefit the wellbeing of staff.

In the hair and beauty industry, you are there to provide a service to clients, so there is not much time to relax and unwind. If you work in a successful salon, you will be rushed off your feet. The area that your employer provides for your rest periods is therefore very important.

The Reporting of Injuries, Diseases and Dangerous Occurrences Regulations 1995 (RIDDOR)

Under these regulations, the employer must send a report to the local authority if:

- anyone dies or is seriously injured at work
- anyone is absent from work for more than three days because of a diagnosed disease or accident connected with work.

Reporting accidents

Although not all accidents must be reported to the local authority, all accidents and injuries must nevertheless be reported to the relevant person. If a workplace employs more than ten staff then by law it must have an accident book. This can be bought from a stationery shop and must be kept somewhere that is easy for all staff to access. The Data Protection Act states that an employee's information must be kept secure and private. Therefore, once the completed sheet is removed from the accident book, it should be passed to the relevant person to be filed in a lockable cabinet. If your salon is small with less than ten employees, it is still a good idea for the employer to keep a record of all accidents and injuries.

ACCIDENT REPORT FORM

SECTION 1 PERSONAL DETAILS

Full name of first aider/staff member: _____

Position held in salon: _____

Date: _____

Accident (injury) ☐ Incident (illness) ☐

Time and date of accident/incident: _____

Full name of injured/ill person: _____

Staff member ☐ Client ☐ Other ☐

Address: _____

Tel. no: _____

SECTION 2 ACCIDENT/INCIDENT DETAILS

Describe what happened. In the case of an accident, state clearly what the injured person was doing: _____

_____

Name and address/tel. no. of witness(es), if any: _____

_____

Action taken

Ambulance called ☐   Taken to hospital ☐   Sent to hospital ☐   First aid given ☐

Taken home ☐   Sent home ☐   Returned to work ☐

SECTION 3 PREVENTATIVE ACTION

Preventative action implemented ☐

Describe action taken: _____

_____

Date implemented: _____

Signature of first aider/staff member: _____

Signature of salon manager/owner: _____

Date: _____

A page from an accident book

The information that should be included when reporting an accident is:

- the date and time it happened
- the place/area
- the type of accident, for example, a cut, a fall or a bang on the head, and how it happened
- the name of the injured or ill person
- what first aid was given, if any
- what happened after the accident – whether the person went to hospital, was sent home or returned to work
- the name and signature of the first aider or person who sorted the matter out.

Top tip

If you need to report an accident, remain calm and think very carefully about what you need to do.

It is not your responsibility to deal with accidents or give first aid. However, you *must* report to your health and safety supervisor anything that you think might be a danger to the general public and staff. So make sure you know who your supervisor is.

Health and safety laws (3)

Always find out the fire and evacuation procedure for any place in which you work or study. By law an employer, school or college must give you this information straight away. If it has not, make sure that you find out as soon as possible.

The Fire Precaution Work Place Regulations 1997

The law says that all workplaces must carry out a **fire risk assessment** and a yearly fire drill. All staff must be trained in the fire drill – what to do in the event of a fire and how to **evacuate** the building safely.

The fire drill

The information that staff should be given about the fire drill includes:

- how to sound the alarm and call for help
- who to report to
- the responsibilities of staff to both clients and the people they work with
- how to leave the building safely
- where the emergency exit is
- where the **assembly point** is.

Your responsibilities at work: fire safety

Do:

- leave all doors unlocked wherever possible
- keep **flammable** products such as aerosols away from heat
- report anything that you think may be a fire **hazard** – it is better to be safe than sorry.

Don't:

- block doorways and exits
- smoke inside
- warm towels on electric or gas heaters.

Building evacuation procedures in the event of fire or bomb alert

The following procedure has been agreed and must be followed. Any staff member who does not comply is committing an infringement of the college disciplinary code. Whenever a fire occurs, the main consideration is to get everybody out of the building safely. Protection of personal or college property is incidental.

Raising the alarm

Anyone discovering a fire must immediately raise the alarm by operating the nearest fire alarm and report to the controller the fire location.

On hearing the alarm the receptionist will immediately contact the emergency services and then evacuate the building.

In the event of a fire being discovered when the reception is unmanned – the premises officer on duty will contact the emergency services and assume control.

On hearing the alarm

All those in senior positions proceed to the control point, normally at a main entrance to the building – where one person must take control of the proceedings.

All other staff: close windows; switch off machinery and lights, and close doors on leaving the room.

Assist less able colleagues, leave the building by the nearest marked route and proceed quickly to the appropriate assembly point. Staff must supervise their class.

Staff evacuating the building must check their locality is clear.

Assembly points

Everyone must remain at assembly points well away from buildings and clear of access roads.

Report to control in person or via two-way radios where allocated.

Everyone must remain at assembly points until further instructions.

DO NOT re-enter the building until you are told it is safe to do so.

An example of a fire evacuation procedure

 Get up and go!

What other responsibilities for fire prevention can you think of? Add some more to the do and don't lists, then write them in a table like the one below. In the second column, write down the reason for each action. In other words, write down the hazards then explain what the risks are.

Hazard	Risk
Blocked doorways and exits	
Smoking inside	
Warming towels on electric heaters	

Fire extinguishers

All workplaces must have fire-fighting equipment which is easy to access and in good working order. All fire extinguishers are colour-coded to indicate the type of fire they can be used for. Before you use a fire extinguisher, you must read the label to make sure you fully understand what type of fire extinguisher it is and what type of fire it is safe to use on. Using a fire extinguisher is not easy and, unless you are confident that you know how and which one to use, don't try – you could put yourself or others at risk.

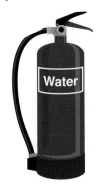 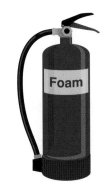 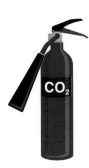 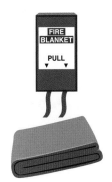 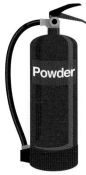

Class A

A water extinguisher can be used to put out fires involving paper, coal, textiles and wood

Class B

A foam extinguisher can be used to put out fires involving **flammable** liquids such as grease, oil, petrol and paints (but not cooking oil or grease)

Class C

A carbon dioxide extinguisher can be used to put out fires involving flammable gases

Class F

A blanket can be used to put out fires involving cooking oils and fats

Class Electrical

A dry powder extinguisher can be used to put out electrical fires

The Electricity at Work Regulations 1989

This law requires that electrical equipment is safe to use and safely maintained. All electrical appliances must be checked regularly. In a busy salon, this may be every six months. These checks must be carried out either by a qualified electrician or a skilled person who is trained and experienced in the use of that particular appliance, for example, a person employed by the company who supplies the equipment.

All electrical checks must be written in a book that is kept specifically for this reason. The date and signature of the person who carried out the check must be entered along with the reason for the check, for example, whether it was a repair or just a maintenance check. Information must be given about the nature of the repair or check.

The book must be available for inspection by the health and safety authority.

Your responsibilities at work: electrical appliances

Report to your supervisor immediately: any faulty plugs, frayed wires or loose connections and any flickering or faulty lights.

Do:

- switch off and unplug all machines after use
- check that all equipment trolleys are stable and not on uneven floors
- wind up wires and cables neatly.

Don't:

- touch electrical equipment, plugs or switches with wet hands or place bowls of water nearby
- leave trailing wires
- plug in or use any equipment that has been reported as faulty.

» Get up and go!

Look for pictures on the Internet of other types of fire-fighting equipment. Cut them out and display them with a brief description of how you would use them and what type of fire they would be used for.

Health and safety laws [4]

The Gas Safety (Installation and Use) Regulations 1994

Under these regulations, a workplace must allow gas and HSE inspectors to enter the **premises** in order to disconnect dangerous gas appliances. All gas appliances must be installed, maintained and used safely.

Your responsibilities at work: gas appliances

Report to your supervisor *immediately*:

- any unusual smell
- any regular headaches, nausea (feeling sick) or unexplained tiredness.

The Manual Handling Operations Regulations 1992

The **Health and Safety Executive** introduced the Manual Handling Operations Regulations in 1992 to prevent injury to the muscles and bones of the body. Injury can be caused by:

- wrong lifting methods
- poor posture
- regular and continual strain on the same part of the body
- moving objects by force that may be too heavy.

Posture, lifting and carrying

In the salon, you need to be careful how you lift and carry stock. You also need to take care over the way you sit, whether at reception or while carrying out a treatment – it is important that the chair or couch is the right height for you. To enable your body to change position regularly while working, it is better if you carry out a variety of treatments. In addition, you need to know how to hold tools correctly, and give your hands a chance to rest after a treatment.

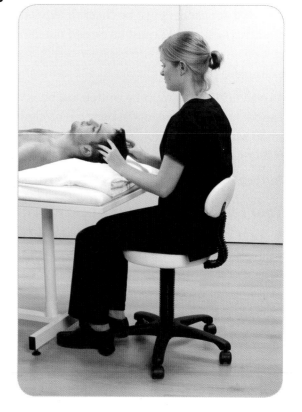

Good posture

Top tips ✓

- If you are unsure about whether you can lift something on your own, always get help.

- If stock needs to be stored on high shelves, make sure you use a safe and stable step ladder – never use a chair.

- Most deliveries are brought to reception. Some are very large and heavy, and will need to be moved elsewhere before they are unpacked. It is very important that large and heavy deliveries are moved carefully to avoid damaging you or the products.

It is a good idea to:

- use height-adjustable couches and cutting stools
- get help when carrying large, heavy or awkward things
- move and stretch your body regularly if you remain in the same position for a long time
- do exercises to keep your hands flexible
- maintain good posture.

Safe lifting method

As a member of staff, you will have a lifetime of bending and standing in one position and it is essential that you look after your back. The safe lifting method is shown below; make sure that you follow it.

When picking up a large or heavy item:

- bend at the knee
- use both hands to grasp the item
- use the strength in your legs to help lift the weight
- never bend from the waist, as this could damage your lower back.

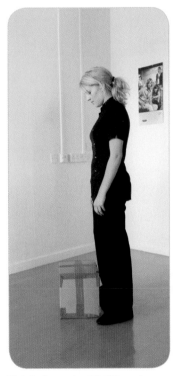 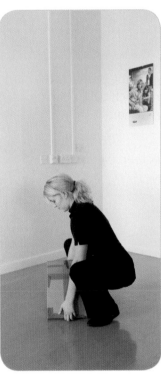 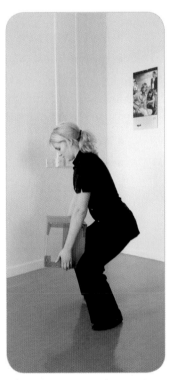 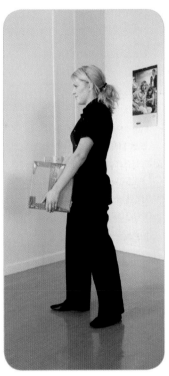

Think about the lift. Where is the load to be placed? Do you need help? Are handling aids available?

With your feet close to the load, bend your knees and keep your back straight. Tuck in your chin. Lean slightly forward over the load to get a good grip.

When you are sure of your grip on the load, straighten your legs and lift smoothly. Remember to keep your back straight.

Carry the load close to your body.

Health and safety laws (5)

The Personal Protective Equipment at Work Regulations 1992

These regulations state that staff must have training in the use of equipment, and details the use of protective clothing for safety at work.

Your responsibilities at work: equipment and clothing

- Never use any equipment for which you have not received training.
- Always wear the recommended protective clothing.

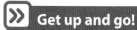

Get up and go!

Ask your tutor which hazardous substances are used on your course. Ask to look at the list that says how they should be handled.

The Control of Substances Hazardous to Health Regulations 2002 (COSHH)

This law requires employers to assess the risks from all harmful products and take appropriate **precautions**. All products that could be harmful must be:

- used safely according to the manufacturer's instructions
- stored safely
- cleaned up safely when spilt
- thrown away safely.

Employers must write down all the products they use, how they are used, stored, cleaned up and thrown away (including cleaning agents). Employers must do this because the products they use could:

Top tip ✓

It is very important that the manufacturer's instructions are followed. These are usually shown on the packaging of a product, or on a separate leaflet inside the box.

- be **flammable**
- be poisonous if swallowed
- cause irritation
- give out strong fumes
- be dangerous if inhaled
- be slippery if spilt.

The simplest way to record information about the different products used by a salon is in a table, which is clear and easy to read. An example is given below.

Product	Hazard	Correct use	Storage	Disposal of waste	Caution
Nail varnish remover	Inhalation of fumes; highly flammable	Replace bottle tops immediately; no smoking or naked flames nearby	Store away from direct heat in a locked cupboard, with lids fully on and bottle upright	Do not dispose of by burning	If spilt, clear up immediately as it can dissolve some plastics such as cushion flooring, and mark trolleys and equipment. If spilt on clothes, minimise the fumes by sponging with water

Manufacturer's instructions

All equipment and products used in a salon must be used in line with the manufacturer's instructions and guidelines. If they are used incorrectly they could cause damage, injury or some other danger to the safety of clients and staff. The instructions also cover the disposal and maintenance of products and equipment. Any accidents or injuries that occur when the manufacturer's instructions are not followed would not be covered by the salon's insurance. It is a legal requirement that all instructions are included with all equipment and products, so it is essential that they are followed.

The Health and Safety Regulations (First Aid) 1981

This act tells employers what they must do to help prevent accidents, and how to deal with accidents when they happen. The employer must follow their rules and guidelines.

The main requirements are:

- a suitably stocked first aid box
- an appointed person to take care of first aid arrangements.

What is first aid?

- First aid is the first help given to someone with an injury or who has become ill. It is the treatment given before the person receives professional medical aid.
- First aid includes calling for help or telephoning for an ambulance (if the problem is serious).

First aid does **not** include:

- giving medicines or tablets
- moving a person who has fallen and could possibly have broken bones – his or her injury could be made worse.

The Health and Safety Regulations (First Aid) 1981 state that there should be a member of staff who is trained in first aid. Once this person has been trained, he or she is qualified for three years. After this time, the person will need to re-train.

It is the job of the first aider to try to prevent a casualty from becoming worse before the ambulance or doctor arrives.

Important things to remember when dealing with a casualty are:

- stay calm
- listen to the person and talk quietly to him or her
- be gentle and caring
- move the casualty as little as possible
- keep the person warm with a blanket, but do not allow him or her to get too hot.

Health and safety laws (6)

The first aid box

A first aid kit must be in a proper first aid box. This is a green box with a white cross on the front. A first aid kit must not be kept in any other type of container, such as a biscuit tin or shoe box.

The first aid box must be kept in a place where all staff can access it easily. It should not be hidden from view and must be labelled clearly.

The first aid box must only contain items that a first aider has been trained to use. It must not contain any medication.

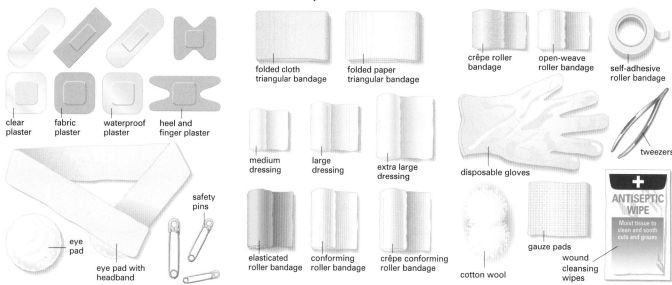

clear plaster • fabric plaster • waterproof plaster • heel and finger plaster

folded cloth triangular bandage • folded paper triangular bandage

crêpe roller bandage • open-weave roller bandage • self-adhesive roller bandage

medium dressing • large dressing • extra large dressing

disposable gloves

tweezers

eye pad • eye pad with headband • safety pins

elasticated roller bandage • conforming roller bandage • crêpe conforming roller bandage

cotton wool

gauze pads

wound cleansing wipes

ANTISEPTIC WIPE — Moist tissue to clean and sooth cuts and grazes

The contents of a first aid box

≫ Get up and go!

Think about the places where you have worked, or your school/college. Find out the following information:

- Where are the first aid boxes kept?
- Do they contain enough of the important first aid items?
- Are the contents checked regularly so that used items are replaced?

Top tip ✓

Don't place tools in your pockets as many are pointed or sharp and could result in an injury if you fall or bump into someone.

The Environmental Protection Act 1990, Waste Regulations 1992 and Special Waste Regulations 1996

These regulations state that clinical waste must be separated from normal waste and disposed of by licensed incineration. Clinical waste means waste items consisting of human tissue, blood, bodily fluids, swabs, dressings, syringes or needles, and incineration means official and permitted burning.

Your responsibilities at work: clinical waste

- Never dispose of clinical waste in a normal waste bin.

The Local Government (Miscellaneous Provisions) Act 1982

Practitioners who carry out a treatment involving the use of needles or skin piercing must register with their local authority. The workplace **premises** also need to be registered, unless the practitioner is mobile, in which case the registration will be for them only. The cost for this registration differs slightly between different authorities.

After the premises or practitioner is registered to carry out the treatments, a local authority inspector will visit to check that the levels of hygiene and safety are satisfactory. Once the checks have been satisfactorily completed, and if the practitioner is qualified, the inspector awards a certificate that allows the following treatments to be carried out:

- acupuncture
- ear and body piercing
- tattooing
- epilation.

 Get ahead

Investigate some more health and safety regulations that are not covered here and that you think may be helpful in the future.

? Memory jogger

1 What does COSHH stand for?

2 What does RIDDOR stand for?

3 What is meant by the term 'clinical waste'?

4 How should you bend when picking up a large or heavy item?

5 When did the Health and Safety Executive introduce the Manual Handling Operations Regulations?

A 1982

B 1992

C 1994

D 2002

6 How would you identify a first aid box?

A White with a green cross

B Green all over

C White all over

D Green with a white cross

7 List three things to remember when dealing with a casualty.

8 Which treatments must be registered under the Local Government (Miscellaneous Provisions) Act 1982?

9 List four responsibilities for electrical safety while at work.

» Get up and go!

Contact your local council for information on the registration of ear piercing, tattooing and epilation in your area.

Workplace policies [1]

Workplace policies and codes of practice

As well as following the Health and Safety at Work Act, your workplace will have its own rules and guidelines for keeping employees and the general public safe. These are called workplace policies or codes of practice.

It is the employer's duty to provide a safe environment for employees. In addition, employees have a duty to co-operate with the workplace policies in order to demonstrate expected standards of behaviour and to make the salon a safer and healthier place to work.

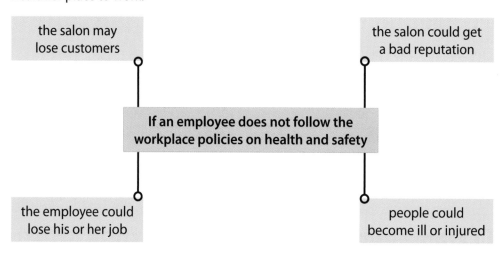

| the salon may lose customers | | the salon could get a bad reputation |

If an employee does not follow the workplace policies on health and safety

| the employee could lose his or her job | | people could become ill or injured |

What are the consequences of not following workplace policies?

 Top tip ✓

It is important that you know who to report hazards, risks, accidents, illnesses and injury to. You will need to make sure that you are familiar with these people at the beginning of your work experience and employment.

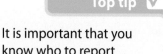 **Get ahead**

Design an information sheet that lists all the important people who are responsible for safety in your salon. For example:

1 The name of the first aider(s) and the days on which they work.

2 The name of the salon manager or supervisor who is generally responsible for help and advice in the salon.

3 The following information about the person in charge of health and safety in your salon: their first name and surname; the days/hours he or she works and who is responsible if that person is away; his or her telephone number and/or place of contact.

 Get up and go!

If you are doing work experience or have a Saturday job, find out your employer's workplace policies and write them down.

Environmentally friendly practices

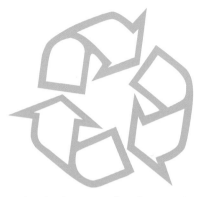

When you are ready to throw packaging out, look at the label to see if it can be recycled

Individuals can make changes in their lifestyles to protect the environment, but the biggest changes will happen when companies and manufacturers take up the necessary changes.

For salons and beauty businesses, it is important to use and buy products made from recycled material where possible as this will increase the demand for recycled products and create a good recycling circle. You can do your bit for the environment while at work, school, college and home. Recycle rubbish such as plastic bottles, jars, paper and card.

When it comes to the working environment, being environmentally friendly is even more important as we use more products and materials and produce much more waste. Your working space and practices must promote environmentally friendly practices. This means that:

- you recycle waste – for example, empty product bottles
- you wash bedding and towels at a lower temperature and wash as much as possible at one time
- you are economical with consumables such as cotton wool and couch roll
- you remember to turn off lighting, heating and hot water heaters when they are not being used
- you don't allow taps to run – it is better to turn them on and off regularly.

Buy Fairtrade goods. Fairtrade is all about better prices and decent working conditions, as well as fair terms of trade for farmers and workers in the developing world.

? Memory jogger

1 What does environmentally friendly mean?
2 List three ways that you should be environmentally friendly at work.
3 What does Fairtrade mean?
4 How can you recycle?

≫ Get up and go!

How many more ways can you think of to be environmentally friendly in the salon environment?

Create an informative poster that you can put on the salon or classroom wall to try to get everyone to think more about being environmentally friendly.

Workplace policies (2)

Salon hygiene

>> Get up and go!

In your college or salon, look at the list of ingredients on the bottles of the products used for cleaning and disinfecting.

A clean, tidy and organised salon is one that will appeal to clients. However, it is not just important to keep things clean and tidy so that the salon looks good. It is also vital in order to control the spread of bacteria that could be a danger to clients and staff. Bacteria spread very easily through the use of dirty tools, for example. Good salon hygiene is therefore a must.

Passing on infection

Infection can pass from one person to another in two ways: direct contact and indirect contact.

- Direct contact is when an infection passes straight from one person to another. This can occur by touching the skin, sneezing, coughing or breathing.
- Indirect contact is when infection passes from one person to another through an unclean object, such as a towel, a jar of cream, tweezers, a wet floor or dirty equipment and tools. This is called **cross-infection**.
- Cross-infection is the transfer of germs and bacteria through poor hygiene.

Preventing cross-infection

There are three ways to make sure that the work environment is clean and germ-free.

Top tip ✓

After washing your hands use a disposable paper towel or hand drier as this is more hygienic than a normal towel.

1 Cleaning

This includes cleaning or washing skin, tools and equipment to promote health by reducing the growth of germs and bacteria. It also removes dust and dirt.

- When cleaning the hands, use liquid soap and paper towels as these are the most hygienic.
- Before any **disinfection** and **sterilisation** (see below), always clean tools and equipment by washing them.
- Chemicals used for cleaning include surface agents (surfactants), alcohols and hypochlorites such as hygiene sprays and gels.

2 Disinfection

Disinfection is a form of cleaning in which surfaces, trolleys and equipment are wiped over with a disinfectant solution.

This reduces the numbers of germs and bacteria to a level that is less harmful to health. Most disinfectant solutions are alcohol- or bleach-based.

For treatments in which the skin must be very clean, such as electrolysis or ear piercing, a disinfectant solution or wipe is used on the skin.

To keep previously sterilised tools (see below) clean during a treatment, place them in a jar of disinfectant solution.

3 Sterilisation

Sterilisation is a cleaning method that kills all germs and bacteria. It is used for tools and equipment. The tools are heated to a very high temperature to kill all germs and bacteria.

However, if the **sterilisation** routine is not thorough, some germs will remain.

There are only two reliable methods of sterilisation:

- dry heat sterilising, which takes place in a hot air oven
- steam sterilising, which takes place in an autoclave.

There are other methods of sterilisation:

- ultraviolet sterilising, which takes place in an ultraviolet cabinet
- heat destruction, which takes place in a bead steriliser.

However, these other methods are not always 100 per cent effective at reaching all the surfaces of the tools. In addition, the temperatures can vary in places, so are not always hot enough to kill the germs and bacteria.

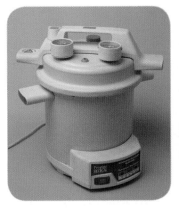

Autoclave

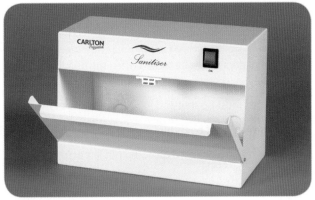

Ultraviolet cabinet

 Top tip

Disinfection and sterilisation are useless on unclean tools and equipment. Your first step must always be to clean them by washing.

Your responsibilities at work: cutting down the risk of infection

1. Wash and dry your hands before and after treating each client.
2. Hold sterilised tools by the handle only.
3. Always use clean towels and a protective couch roll for each client.
4. Wipe down surfaces and trolleys with a disinfectant solution regularly.
5. Keep your nails short with no varnish, and tie your hair back neatly.
6. Don't share tools.
7. Remove all jewellery.
8. Use disposable tools where possible.
9. Wear a clean and fresh uniform.
10. Re-sterilise any tools that have been dropped on the floor.
11. Wear a plaster on any cuts or grazes.
12. Replace tops on products straight away.
13. Don't eat and drink in the salon area.
14. Always use spatulas to remove creams from jars.
15. Never cough, sneeze or blow your nose over a client.
16. Dust and clean the work area regularly.
17. Don't carry out a treatment if you have a cold or the 'flu.
18. Never treat open cuts, bites or stings.
19. Use sterilised equipment only.
20. Never treat anyone with who has a contra-indication (you can find more information about this in units B2, B3 and N1).

Workplace policies (3)

Security and safekeeping

The security of takings, staff, clients and their belongings is important in a salon. No one wants their belongings lost and your employer does not want hard-earned money lost, or worse, stolen. In this section, you will learn about how to protect the workplace, clients and products from theft.

At the salon

A salon owner needs to make sure that the business **premises** are secure. The salon will not be covered by insurance for fire, theft or damage if it is not. It is therefore vital that the correct steps are carried out to secure the building.

When closed:	When open:
All external doors must be locked when the building is empty.	Senior members of staff should bank money regularly.
All windows must be shut and locked at the end of the day.	
Burglar alarms must be turned on.	There should be a secure safe for money that cannot be banked until later in the day.
All money must be banked daily and not left on the premises or in the till.	
The till must be emptied at the end of the day and left open.	There should be an electronic till, which is used by one or two members of staff only.
A security nightlight should be installed, to deter burglars.	
A trustworthy person, either a member of staff or a neighbour, should be given a spare key in case of emergency; the person's name and address should be given to the police.	All visitors must be checked in at reception.

Health and Safety at Work Act 1974

Within this act it states that all employers must provide a safe system of cash handling. For example, if an employee is sent to the bank to pay money in alone and is then robbed or mugged, the employer could be prosecuted.

Staff and clients

To avoid loss, theft or damage of goods and valuables that belong to staff and clients, lockers should be provided for valuables and handbags. Staff should avoid bringing valuables or large sums of money to work and clients should keep their handbags and valuables with them at all times, unless client lockers are available in the salon. Clients should themselves place jewellery or valuables in their handbag, or keep such items in full view during a treatment.

Stock

To protect stock against theft, the stock cupboard should remain locked and the key kept in a safe place, preferably in the office. One or two senior members of staff should be responsible for giving out stock for treatments and refilling of products, and products for retail should be kept in full view of the reception desk in a locked display cabinet. The key for the cabinet should be placed on a hook behind the reception

Top tip ✓

As a trainee, it is not your responsibility to take money to the bank for paying in or to handle large amounts of money.

desk, where it cannot be seen or reached by visitors. If a locked cabinet is not available for displaying products, the empty boxes should be put on display and the products kept in the locked stock cupboard. Finally, you should carry out weekly stock checks to make sure that the amounts of stock match with what should be there.

Insurance

Employer's Liability (Compulsory Insurance) Act 1969

This insurance is compulsory for employers and business owners. All employees, clients and visitors to the salon must be covered under this insurance in case they injure themselves or catch a disease at work. The certificate of insurance must be displayed in the workplace for all to see. It will include the following details:

- the name of the business and owner
- the type of business
- the start date and end date of the insurance
- the name of the insurance company.

Your employer may also have professional indemnity insurance. This covers claims against employees if they cause injury or damage to a client or client's property through their irresponsible actions and behaviour. (If an employee does not take out this insurance, they must make sure that they are fully covered on the employer's liability insurance.)

If the salon building is rented or leased the property owner is responsible for insuring it against fire or damage. However, if the building is owned by the salon, the salon owner will need to take out buildings insurance. Finally, the contents of the business will need to be insured against accidental damage, fire or theft. Contents insurance covers items such as tools, equipment, furniture, products and valuables, although this insurance will not cover damage caused through **negligence** or natural wear and tear.

>> **Get up and go!**

Check out how many insurance liability certificates you can see in different shops, offices and businesses that you go into. Every business, including beauty salons, must have these displayed so that people can see them. How many are you able to see?

? **Memory jogger**

1 Who or what does employer's liability insurance protect?
   A Employers
   B Staff and visitors
   C Buildings
   D Business contents
2 What is professional indemnity insurance?
3 What insurance is compulsory for employers and business owners?

Personal presentation and behaviour

A high standard of presentation and hygiene at work is necessary in order to follow the salon guidelines and communicate the salon's image as a clean and professional place of business. It will also give clients a good impression of you, as well as making you feel more confident.

Personal hygiene

You must always take care to ensure good personal hygiene at work.

Action	How it improves personal hygiene
Bath or shower daily	To remove stale sweat, which will begin to smell as bacteria grows in it
Use an underarm anti-perspirant or deodorant daily	To keep you smelling fresh and to cut down on sweating
Step up your mouth hygiene! Look after your teeth and gums: ■ clean your teeth twice daily ■ floss daily ■ rinse with a mouthwash while at work	Clean teeth and gums mean fresh breath. If you continue to have a mouth odour problem, you could have a build-up of old food around your teeth and gums A mouthwash will help to keep your mouth fresh and stop bacteria from growing in your mouth
Wear a clean, ironed uniform	Uniforms can easily become dirty and absorb smells in the environment, including smells from other people and body odour
Have short, neat nails with no varnish	Dirt, germs and bacteria build up under long nails. Varnish-free nails look cleaner and fresher than painted ones. Some clients can be sensitive to the ingredients in nail varnish
Wash your hands with soap and dry them thoroughly after every visit to the toilet	If you do not wash and dry your hands thoroughly, you may pass many bacteria and germs to others when you carry out a treatment
Never eat in the salon area	Eating in the salon area causes the spread of bacteria and will encourage the presence of insects and disease-spreading flies
Remove jewellery when carrying out a treatment	Bacteria can build up under rings

Your personal presentation is very important

Personal conduct

Conducting yourself positively and behaving in the right way is something that you will need to do throughout your working life. Positive behaviour ranges from demonstrating good body language and good posture, to fair treatment and respect of others along with a willingness to learn.

Your salon will have policies for behaviour and good conduct and these must be followed at all times, otherwise you could risk your job or work experience placement. Salons, as with all public places, must be a non-smoking environment, but remember that even if staff have a cigarette outside during a break, the smell remains on their clothes and breath and can be smelt by clients during their treatment. An alcohol- and drug-free workplace is also essential. Any member of staff under the influence of drugs or alcohol cannot use equipment and products safely and could put others at risk. If clients are under the influence of drugs or alcohol, they will be asked to leave by the supervisor or relevant person.

 Salon life

Karen was going to do her work experience at Vitality and Vitesse. Although she thought the salon looked great, Lindy, her manager, was strict and seemed obsessed with the appearance of her staff when she interviewed Karen.

Karen was only there for two weeks so didn't have the usual staff uniform, but was allowed to wear black trousers and a black t-shirt and flat shoes. On her first day, Lindy looked over Karen's workwear and told her that her trousers were too long and frayed at the edges, her t-shirt was too short and showed off her tummy and pierced navel and that her peep-toe shoes were too high. Karen said that this was all she had at home and her mum couldn't afford to buy her new clothes and shoes just for the two weeks. Lindy explained that she had made the dress code very clear at the interview. Karen then had to work in the laundry room on her first day and Lindy said that she would arrange a spare uniform for the following day.

Karen washed, tumbled and ironed her way throughout the day as well as fetching and carrying up and down the stairs for the therapists. At 12 o'clock Janice, the apprentice, dropped a pair of scissors and they fell right on Karen's toes poking out from her peep-toe shoes. Later she was asked to carry some fresh towels upstairs with Suki but on the way up the stairs, Suki trod on her long, frayed trousers and Karen fell over. Luckily, she wasn't badly hurt, just shaken up, and after a cup of tea she went back to ironing some duvet covers for the couches. She didn't concentrate, though, and leant on the iron, which burnt her bare tummy. That really was the last straw for Karen and she burst out crying and stormed out of the salon.

Why is it important to present yourself properly?

What could happen if you try to bend the rules about dress code and behaviour?

 Get ahead

Research your workplace's code of conduct. Why do you think it has each rule? What would be the consequences of not following the rules?

? Memory jogger

1 Why are good personal presentation and conduct important at work?

2 Why should you remove jewellery before carrying out a treatment?

Getting ready for assessment

What you must cover during your practical assessments

Safe, healthy and hygienic working practices should be something that you demonstrate throughout all of your practical treatments. It should not be something that you follow just to pass an assessment. For example, when you are being assessed carrying out a practical task you will be able to cover G20 performance criteria and your assessor will be able to sign you off for different areas each time.

Carrying out a practical treatment using unhygienic tools, or without carrying out a risk assessment of your work area to avoid accidents happening, will mean that you are not safe to do a treatment and therefore could mean that you do not pass your assessment.

What you must know

In order to pass this unit you will need to know about information and regulations that are relevant to health and safety. You will gather evidence on this during classwork and further study and will probably file it in a portfolio of evidence. This evidence will also be signed off in your candidate log book, which you will be given by your assessor. This will be an official record to show that you have covered what you need to.

Top tips ☑

- Before using any products or equipment read the manufacturer's instructions and follow any previous instructions given to you by your assessor.
- Keep a look out for any unsafe practices.
- Report any hazards to your assessor immediately.

Salon life

Maz had been working at the Green Rooms for three weeks and although she enjoyed it she found it a nuisance that there were so many rules and regulations that the staff had to follow. She felt it really wasn't necessary; the list of rules seemed endless, and she kept getting into trouble for the slightest thing. For example, yesterday she threw out some empty product bottles and was told that they could be used again. The day before she got told off for using too much cotton wool and tissue, and the day before that she left some bottle tops off and her manager got really cross. The previous week she felt really cold but had forgotten her work cardigan, so shut the windows and turned off the air conditioning – yes, you can guess, she got into trouble for that as well.

What were the things that Maz did wrong and why do you think they were wrong?

What could happen if everyone constantly did the things that Maz had done?

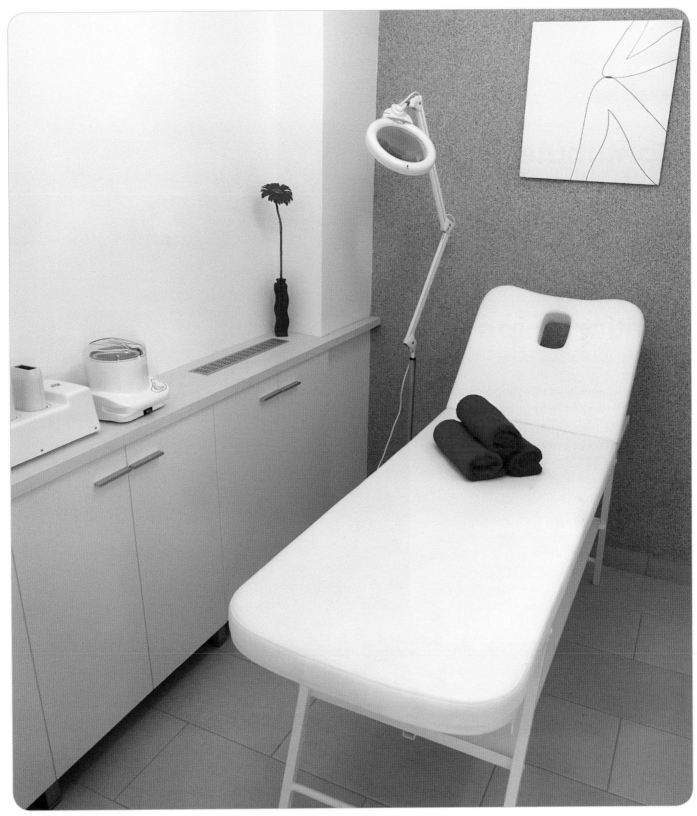

The salon is a fantastic place to work, but you must make
sure that you follow health and safety regulations

UNIT G3

Contribute to the development of effective working relationships

During your career in hairdressing or beauty therapy you will need to form and maintain good working relationships with clients and colleagues. If positive working relationships are not maintained, this could result in an unhappy atmosphere at work, lack of trust and a drop in clientele.

Effective working relationships will help you to enjoy your work, and if all members of the team work together the running of a business is like finding all of the pieces of the jigsaw puzzle. If one piece falls apart many things within the business will suffer or fail.

In this unit you will learn how to:

- Develop effective working relationships with clients
- Develop effective working relationships with colleagues
- Develop yourself within your job role.

Here are some key terms you may meet in this unit:

Scripts –
set lists of words to use

Aggression –
anger, annoyance or loss of temper

Commission –
a small percentage of the price of a product that is given to the person who sells it

Target –
aim, ambition, purpose

Overtime –
extra work beyond your normal working hours

Tactless remarks –
remarks made without any thought or consideration as to how they will annoy or upset the person who hears them

Adapt –
change in order to meet different needs

Anticipate –
expect, wait for

Resentment –
dislike, bitterness or anger

Prioritising –
putting the most important things first

Grievance –
cause to complain

Personal development plan –
a plan of how you will develop your job role and career

Promotion –
moving up to a more senior job

Trade journals –
magazines for the industry

Confidence –
when you have a positive feeling or opinion about someone or something

Develop effective working relationships with clients [1]

A salon builds its reputation on how satisfied clients and visitors are. If clients leave the salon unhappy, angry and upset, the word soon spreads to other people and bookings for treatments and services will fall. This means that building effective working relationships with your clients is vital to the successful running of the business. Being a hairdresser can be very much like being an actress at times; even when you aren't feeling very happy yourself you must not let this show. The client is spending money to feel good and you will be expected to do your best to help their visit go well. As you spend your working day attending to and treating clients, being able to develop good relationships with them will also help to increase the enjoyment that you get from your work.

Appearance and hygiene

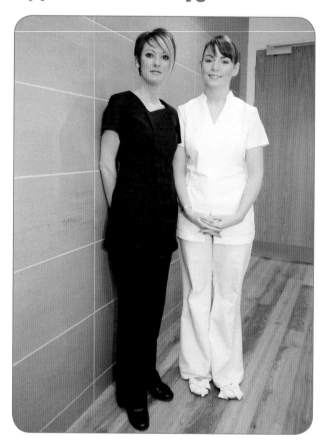

You must always look professional

How you look and behave will obviously affect how your clients feel about their experience in your salon. Looking professional and behaving professionally will help to give your clients **confidence** in you.

Your salon will have rules about appearance and you will be told how you must present yourself and, whether you think it is fashionable or not, you must follow what you are told. You must make sure that you are freshly showered each day and that you have clean, fresh breath.

Uniform

All salons have their own style and how they want their staff to look. Some salons prefer white whereas others prefer black or colour. The uniforms could be dresses, tunics and skirts, or tunics and trousers.

Whatever you are expected to wear as part of the salon's look, it must be clean, ironed and hemmed and without any buttons missing or broken zips. The smallest dip in standards of appearance will be noticed by your supervisor and the clients and you would be letting yourself down as well as them. Shoes must usually be low heeled and enclosed for health and safety reasons.

The other reason why uniform is worn is for protection while you work. This comes under the Personal Protective Equipment at Work Regulations, which was covered on page 20.

Hair

Hair must usually be tied up, making sure there is no loose hair around your face and neck that could dangle on a client's skin when doing a treatment. It must also be very clean and most definitely not smell of smoke.

Jewellery

Small earrings that don't hang are acceptable, as well as a watch, but otherwise all other jewellery should be removed.

Behaviour

You must act in a professional manner at all times when in the salon. Having the right attitude is important no matter who you are working with, whether it is your supervisor, other colleagues or clients.

Your employer will have certain standards for behaviour, and there may be a list of rules. Make sure that you are aware of them all and that you follow them. Failing to follow rules could mean that you lose your job, but making sure that you follow your salon's standards will help you to develop effective relationships at work, as well as making sure that you, your clients and your colleagues remain as safe as possible at all times.

Always follow these basic rules.

- Talk properly without use of slang.
- Turn off mobile phones and don't text friends.
- Don't gossip or chat during work hours.
- Maintain good posture, as slouching around looks as though you don't care.
- Don't shout across a room – go over and talk quietly instead.
- Don't smoke on the premises or in view of clients outside the building.
- Don't eat or drink except in the staff room.

 Get up and go!

Record three examples of people on the telephone, either making appointments or answering enquiries (you could do this on your mobile phone). Then let the rest of the class hear and ask them to decide who they think sounds the best and the most professional. Ask for ideas as to how the others could be improved.

Develop effective working relationships with clients (2)

Communication

The key to all good relationships, whether personal, business or work relationships, is effective communication. There are many different forms of communication, but all are built on our ability to pass on information, feelings and understanding through speaking, writing or body language.

Different methods of communication include:

- Oral communication – speaking to another person. This includes speaking by telephone or face-to-face conversations.
- Written communication – for example, letters, memos, faxes, text messages and email.
- Body language – for example nodding, smiling and making eye contact.
- Images – communicating information through adverts, posters, magazines and brochures.

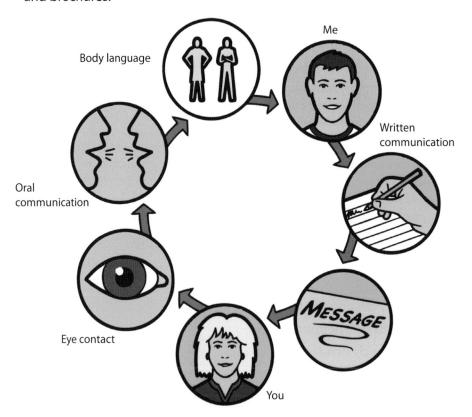

Methods of communication

Positive and negative communication

As we have seen, communication does not just mean what you say out loud. You also communicate with people through the way in which you use words and your body language. It is important that all of the messages that you communicate are positive ones.

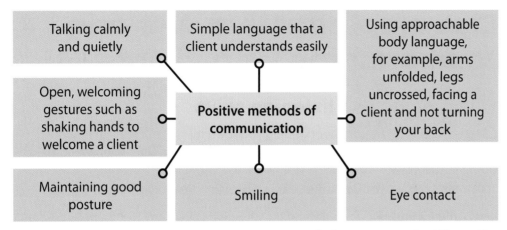

All of your messages should be positive

Sometimes, if you are not feeling great, it can be hard to make sure that you use only positive methods of communication. However, no matter how you are feeling, the use of negative methods will not be a successful way to get your message or point across.

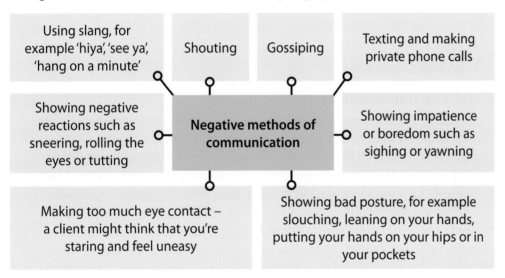

Negative methods of communication are not a good way to express yourself

Always pay attention to your body language as you might communicate a negative message to a client or colleague, for example that you are bored, without really meaning to. These negative methods are all barriers to communication and should never be used at work. Think about how you would react if someone used these negative methods with you.

In order to show a good image of yourself and the salon to clients, and to maintain good relationships with your colleagues, you must communicate clearly, politely and confidently. Clients need to feel that they can trust you and that you will maintain their confidentiality.

Develop effective working relationships with clients (3)

Questioning and listening skills

Communicating is not just about getting your own message across – it is about understanding, interpreting and reacting to messages that other people might be giving you, and also about asking questions.

Good questioning skills will help you to find out about:

- job roles and responsibilities
- a person's personality
- how a client or colleague may be feeling.

Quite often people ask questions without really listening to the answer. This is not a good way to communicate and you could miss valuable information such as:

- how a colleague or client is
- what a client wants from a treatment or service
- what your boss expects of you.

Good and bad questioning techniques

In the hair and beauty industry, you will need to communicate with clients when giving client consultations, advice and aftercare, and when selling products and treatments. You will also need to build good relationships with clients and colleagues and pass on important information. You therefore need to make sure not only that you speak clearly, but also that your style of communicating and questioning is appropriate.

Consultations are question-and-answer sessions that are designed to find out information about a client. You should use positive methods of communication including listening skills and give them time to speak before interrupting them. Below are some examples of good and bad questioning techniques: good questioning uses open questions that allow a full answer, whereas bad questioning techniques use closed questions that result in a 'Yes' or 'No' answer.

- Good: 'Tell me about your hair and skin care routine at home.'
- Bad: 'Do you cleanse, tone and moisturise at home?'

Recognising a client's moods

Knowing when a client is happy, annoyed or confused is important. If you are unable to recognise different moods or mood changes in a client you will have no idea what is wrong with them and how you might put it right.

Here are some typical signals that may tell you a client is not happy.

- Huffing – may suggest she is fed up with with being kept waiting.
- Tutting – may suggest that she is annoyed.
- A grumpy expression – could mean she is not enjoying her treatment.
- Tapping her fingers on a surface – may suggest that you are running late.

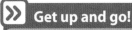
Get up and go!

Think of some positive questions that could be used during a consultation and then think of an opposite, negative one for each to demonstrate the difference.

Get up and go!

In pairs, one of you should imagine that you are unhappy with a service and give non-oral signs to suggest that you are fed up. Your partner should watch carefully and read your body language.

The client's facial expression can also tell you if they are confused. Look out for:

- one eyebrow higher than the other
- a wrinkled nose and crease between the eyebrows
- a raised corner of the mouth.

Another sign may be that they keep asking you to explain the same thing or question you about the same thing, which suggests that they have not received a good enough answer or an answer that is easy to understand.

Rules and procedures

Salon businesses usually have set communication methods and procedures that they expect employees to follow. Some even have set **scripts** that employees need to follow. These may include how to answer the phone, re-book appointments and carry out client consultations.

It is very important that you follow these procedures because they are part of the business's identity and ensure that all staff are following a set of guidelines for communicating with clients, visitors and each other.

Client care

A salon builds its reputation on how satisfied clients are. Many salons will have guidelines for client care and these may include some of the following procedures.

Handling client belongings

When a client removes her coat or removes jewellery, let her see where you are putting it for safekeeping so that she knows where it is. Fold her clothes with care or hang them up and place her jewellery in a bowl that she can see easily. It is better to give it to the client for safekeeping, though. At the end of the treatment, pass her coat and the bowl of jewellery stating what you are doing so that there is no confusion.

Referring client concerns

If at any time your client is worried or has a question that you are unable to answer, you must refer this promptly to a senior member of staff.

Maintaining client comfort and care

Pay attention to client comfort and care before, during and after their treatment. Before the treatment:

- greet them and collect them from reception
- use positive communication and body language.

During the treatment:

- check that they are warm, comfortable and relaxed
- maintain positive communication.

After the treatment:

- check their satisfaction with the treatment
- offer to help them with their coat and belongings
- offer to book their next appointment
- take them back to reception and say goodbye.

> **? Memory jogger**
>
> 1 List three types of positive communication.
> 2 List three types of negative communication.
> 3 What is the difference between an open and a closed question?

Develop effective working relationships with colleagues [1]

Working with other people in a salon is not always easy. It can be necessary for very different personalities to work together in a small environment. Being helpful and supportive while making a positive contribution to the team effort will help you to achieve success with both your workmates and your manager.

You won't necessarily always have great relationships with your colleagues at work. You will need to accept that everyone you work with is different. You are not expected to like all your colleagues, no matter how hard you may try, but you must be able to get along with them. This means that you must respect each other's differences and build good working relationships.

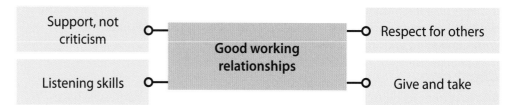

Factors contributing to good working relationships

Teamwork

Teamwork simply means working with others or working together to reach a common goal. At work, staff often work in teams to carry out roles and responsibilities: two heads can often be better than one.

Teamwork is about thinking how you can support the business and colleagues.

- Make yourself useful – keep yourself busy.
- Be available – don't disappear into the staffroom at every opportunity.
- Be ready and willing to assist, this is a key part to your role.
- Try to **anticipate** needs of colleagues and clients, for example by preparing work areas, tools and equipment and products before they have to ask.
- Always wear a smile and be ready to help.

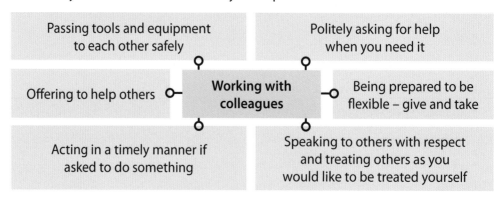

What you need to do when working with colleagues

Top tips

- Teamwork also means sharing work – not necessarily doing the same job, but sharing workloads relating to common tasks.

- There are always jobs to do that are less popular than others, or times when staff are needed to do **overtime**. Don't let it always be the same people who put in the extra effort. If that person is always you, you should be prepared to say 'no' and suggest a fairer system. If you always sneak off when jobs need doing, ask yourself, 'Am I being fair?'

Salon life

Since Debbie and Terry started work at the local salon, they found it difficult to agree on anything. Debbie found Terry very bossy, even though they were both assistants.

It all came to a head on Saturday afternoon. The day had been very busy and very long, and Debbie was sick of Terry ordering her about. 'Tidy this up', 'Have you washed up?', 'Go and work on reception', 'Change the music' – the list was endless. Who did he think he was?

When Terry told Debbie to sweep the reception area Debbie snapped and started shouting at him and told him she was sick of him being so bossy and then told him to sweep up himself! The reception area went deathly quiet and the clients waiting for treatments looked shocked and uncomfortable. Trish, the salon manager, ordered Debbie into the office.

Who was in the wrong – Debbie or Terry?

What could have been done to stop the situation getting this bad?

What could Debbie have done instead of losing her temper?

Get ahead

Find out the differences between aggressive, assertive and passive behaviour in the workplace. Then observe your colleagues or classmates while they are working in a practical session and make notes on whether you think each of them demonstrates aggressive, assertive or passive behaviour and the reasons why.

Present this information as a PowerPoint presentation and deliver your findings to the group with opportunity for discussion afterwards.

Develop effective working relationships with colleagues (2)

Communicating with colleagues

Working effectively with your colleagues will include exchanging different types of information with them and using positive methods of communication. This is just as important when you are working with colleagues as it is when you are working with clients.

Some subjects might be difficult to bring up, such as if you need to tell a colleague that you are unhappy about something they have done or if you need to report a problem to your manager/supervisor, but this means that you need to take even more care to communicate positively.

To work successfully as part of a team you need to listen to other people's views even though you may not agree with them. When you want to put an important point across, you should speak in a calm voice without showing **aggression**. There is more chance that you will be taken seriously and listened to if you don't get angry or lose your temper. Making **tactless remarks** could hurt or offend people. Remember, there is always room for different views and opinions.

It is important to report any information you have been given to the appropriate person straight away, or if this is not possible a note should be left for them. If a colleague needs to know something so that they can carry out their job or deal with a client properly, this information must not be left until later as it could affect how the salon runs.

Respect

You need to have respect for your colleagues to ensure good staff relations. Problems that come up should be discussed immediately. If they are not talked about, **resentment** may build up and this will lead to a bad atmosphere that will spill over into your work. This negative atmosphere may be picked up by clients and other staff members, affecting the salon as a whole.

It is also a good idea to build relationships with other members of staff by checking anything with them that may affect them or their work. If you don't, this could lead to bad feeling and cause conflict. Try to be fair to others and respect their views, methods and belongings.

> **Top tip** ✓
>
> To run successfully, a salon relies on timely reporting of information.

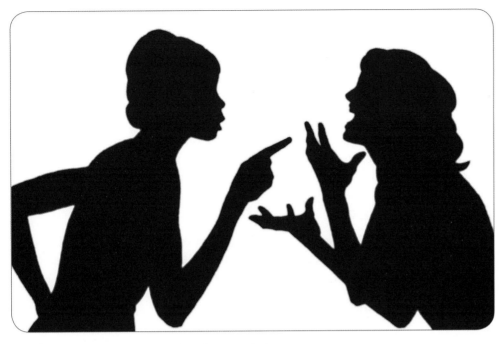

A negative atmosphere will affect the salon as a whole

» Get up and go!

Write a short script in pairs that demonstrates good and bad examples of working relationships and perform this as a role play to the rest of the group.

Reporting difficulties in working with others

At some point in your career you will have difficulties with other colleagues. This could be as simple as a disagreement, but could go from bad to worse if you do not refer problems to a senior member of staff. It is not about telling tales but instead it is about trying to work out any difficulties that you have so that you stay professional and keep the workplace a calm and happy place to work in.

» Get up and go!

Describe the 'ideal' working colleague using a spidergram (there is an example of a spidergram on page 42).

Summary

As a team we should:

- support one another
- watch out for each other
- work well with each other
- communicate well with each other.

? Memory jogger

1 Why is it important to communicate well with colleagues?

2 What could happen if the staff in a salon didn't work as a team?

3 Why must you treat your colleagues with respect?

Develop yourself within your job role (1)

As a Level 1 student you are at the beginning of an exciting career in hairdressing or beauty therapy. It is really important that from the start of your employment you are clear about what your role involves, what your salon expects of you and what your limits of authority are so that you know how to do your job properly. You also need to consider the importance of how to develop yourself within your role so that you can move on from Level 1 to the next step in your beauty therapy career.

Finding out about your job

As discussed in Unit G20 Make sure your own actions reduce risks to health and safety, the legal requirements that salons have play a large part in their success and reputation. As well as this all salons have their own rules and regulations.

Contract of employment

When you get a job you will have a contract of employment. This will cover all sorts of things such as:

- hours you work
- holidays per year
- pension schemes

- disciplinary and **grievance** procedures
- sick pay
- your job role and responsibilities.

Induction

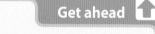

Get ahead

Imagine that you are a salon reception manager.

What things would you cover in your reception induction for new staff?

How would you make sure that your induction had worked?

In addition to receiving your contract of employment, you will also have an induction when you first start a new job or attend work experience. This can be carried out on a one-to-one basis or, if a few new employees are starting at the same time, it may be carried out in a group.

This induction will cover the important information that you need to know about your job, the roles you have and your responsibilities. For example:

- who you report to
- what you must do each day
- health and safety

- members of the staff
- the time you start and finish work
- standards of appearance and behaviour.

Without an induction you would not know what you can and cannot do, what to do if there was an emergency and who you will be working with. It is a large part of your role as a beauty therapy assistant to find out about your salon's requirements and what they will expect of you.

As well as this you will be expected to keep up to date with things about your job. New methods, rules and procedures may be introduced or improvements made to ones already in place. See the information on continuous professional development on page 52 for advice on how to make sure you keep up to date with new developments in the beauty therapy industry.

Attendance and punctuality

Employers expect their staff to have a good attendance record. Staff who take lots of time off can cause difficulties for the business and their colleagues. Not only will the business be short staffed and unable to book as many clients during that time, but the other employees will have to work harder to make up for the person who is away, which puts extra pressure on them at work.

Everyone is ill at some point and this cannot be helped, but it is the people who are continually absent from work that can cause problems for others.

Just as frustrating is the employee who is always late. This means that the day starts badly, things are not prepared, colleagues have to cover until the person eventually arrives and clients can be kept waiting.

Seeking permission

Being employed as an assistant is the first rung on a ladder to a career in the hair/beauty industry and this means that you will always need to get permission from your supervisor before doing anything more than what you have been told to do. This is to make sure that you, your colleagues and your clients stay safe. Make sure that you are aware of your limits of authority and that you do not overstep them.

Reporting difficulties

A range of difficulties may come up during your working day. These could include:

- problems with another colleague
- too much work to do and not enough time
- not understanding instructions and needing further help
- a mistake that you have made.

It is important to report any difficulty that you are unable to deal with to someone more senior, no matter how small it is, as small problems can become large ones if ignored.

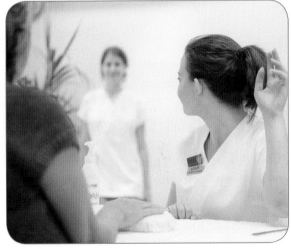

Make sure that you report any difficulties you come across

Salon grievance and appeals procedures

Each salon should have a **grievance** and appeals procedure. This may be a simple document that includes information on things such as what to do if you feel that you are being treated unfairly, for example:

- workplace bullying
- being expected to work outside your normal working hours constantly
- being expected to do jobs that you are not qualified to do
- disagreements with others that cannot be sorted out
- working conditions.

It is important that you know about the salon's staffing structure so that you know who is responsible for what and who you need to ask or discuss things with. If you felt that you were being treated unfairly, you should report this to your named supervisor.

 Get ahead

Research on the Internet and find out more about grievance and appeals procedures in the workplace.

Develop yourself within your job role (2)

Procedures and targets

For the salon to be successful, the business and the staff need set procedures and **targets**. Having manageable targets gives everyone something to aim for, especially when a reward is offered if targets are met. A good business recognises this and offers its staff extras on top of their wages if they meet targets and prove themselves to be valuable employees.

Business development targets

Salon businesses set targets for their staff to achieve. This is because they need them to boost the takings and success of the business. Quite often the salon will give their staff an incentive to meet the targets. Targets could be selling products, promoting new treatments or having a busy column.

An incentive could be a **commission** on sales and treatments. This means that staff receive a small percentage of the sales and treatments over and above their normal wages. A typical method might be 10 per cent of the money taken from sales.

Therefore, if you earn £150 per week and sell £50 worth of products in a week, your wages would work out at:

£150 + 10% of £50 (£5) = £155.

Personal development targets

Personal effectiveness in your work role involves aiming all the time to improve your performance. It is based on lots of different things, such as how successfully you communicate, your willingness to do the job, your attitude and how supportive you are to others.

Your personal performance can be developed as you learn a new job and gain new skills. An important framework for this is a **personal development plan**. Creating a personal development plan involves setting personal targets related to your training and career. These are usually based around your performance at work, and your future career aims and plans, such as training and **promotion**.

Setting targets related to these will involve identifying your strengths and weaknesses. Being aware of these will help you to focus on building on what you are good at and improving on what you are not so good at.

Weaknesses are often due to a lack of knowledge and experience and can often be improved with training and experience. For example, you may think that your reception skills are weak, but this may be because you lack **confidence** with clients and experience at the tasks involved in running a reception. With practice and training your confidence will grow and your weaknesses can eventually become your strengths.

Get ahead ⬆

Work out what each member of staff would take home in pay at the end of a week, based on a 10 per cent **commisssion** rate:

- If Claire earns £165 and sells £75 worth of products, how much will her wages be?
- If Matt earns £100 as an apprentice and sells £160 worth of products, how much will his wages be?

Use the table below as a fun way of gaining a clearer picture of the type of person you are. Identify the qualities you think you have from those listed in the table below, and give an example of how you show each quality.

≫ Get up and go!

Quality	Personal example	Quality	Personal example
Punctual		Often late	
A good listener		Doesn't pay attention to others or interrupts	
Uncompetitive		Competitive	
Laid back, never feels rushed		Always in a rush	
Patient, particularly with waiting		Impatient, hates to wait	
Concentrates on one thing at a time – unable to multi-task		Able to multi-task, often taking on too many things	
Slow, deliberate talker		Exuberant, fast talker	
Able to motivate self without the need for praise		Needs constant praise and recognition	
Slow-paced		Does everything at a fast pace, even walking, eating and talking	
Relaxed and easy-going		Tense and stressed	
Expresses feelings		Hides feelings	
Lots of outside interests		Few interests – hard to find the time or energy	
Unambitious		Ambitious, driven	

Once you have identified your strengths and weaknesses in terms of your work, you need to discuss these with your tutor or supervisor at work, and have them agreed. You then need to set some targets and deadlines for achieving those targets and record these, with your supervisor, on your **personal development plan**. It is important that your targets are realistic.

Continually using your personal development plan and updating it as necessary will provide your learning at work with a structure. Working towards meeting your personal targets will help you to grow as a valuable employee and will motivate you to progress on to the next step in your career.

Here are some possible targets that you might set yourself:

- short term (three months) – to pass ten assessments
- medium term (nine months) – to pass all assessments and gain the NVQ Level 1 Diploma in Hairdressing and Beauty Therapy
- long term (three years) – to gain Level 2 or Level 3

Meeting your targets has a number of positive benefits to you. These include respect from others, a sense of satisfaction, promotion and wage improvement.

? Memory jogger

1 How can setting targets help you?

2 When you receive an amount of extra money in your wages from salon sales and treatments, this is called:

A An incentive

B Commission

C Personal development

D A percentage

Develop yourself within your job role (3)

Reviews and feedback

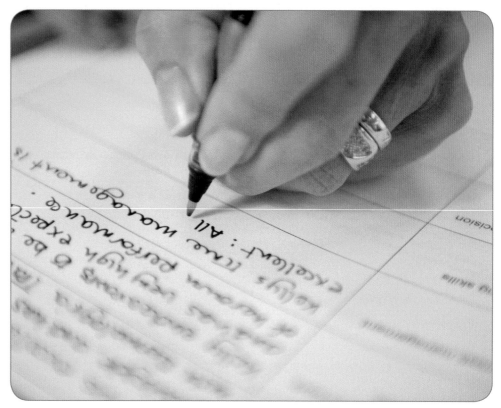

An appraisal form

An important part of improving your performance and developing yourself within your job role is reviewing your progress on a regular basis, both by yourself, with your colleagues and with your employer or tutor. Part of working with others is being able to accept feedback and reviews. Your supervisor will give you feedback on your work regularly. This is not meant to be critical, but is a positive process aimed at improving your performance and helping you to meet your targets. You will need to listen and not take offence.

As well as regular feedback during your career, you will have official reviews called appraisals. These are a formal opportunity for you and your boss to discuss your progress and how you both think you are doing, and for you both to assess whether or not you have met your targets. Did you meet all of your targets within the time scale you set? If not, why not? What did you do well? Are there any areas where you had particular difficulties or where you need more specific training?

You will be able to use the feedback from your appraisal, both on your achievements and on the areas that you need to develop, to set yourself new targets for your future **personal development plan** and to help you progress to the next step in your career.

Taking personal responsibility for your own development

Remember that how well you do at work and how fast you progress is largely down to you. It is important to take responsibility for your own development. If you feel that you have not been given clear enough instructions when you have been asked to do a task, make sure that you ask the relevant person as soon as possible. If you don't ask, you might not be told. If you find a part of your work difficult, ask your supervisor to help you. Remember they all started off as assistants and trainees too.

If you are given opportunities to learn, take advantage of them. Take part as actively as possible in all of the training and development activities you have the chance to be involved in, and take an active role in salon activities. Watch your more senior colleagues perform technical treatments and learn from them.

Managing your time

So that you can manage your time successfully, you need to know what your goals are so that you can plan your time. For example, if your boss has given you a list of jobs to do, you will need to work out how much time you have got to do them in so that you can decide which ones are the most important. This is called **prioritising**.

If you don't learn to manage your time, you may not get the things done that you need to and could become stressed. Things that you will need to time-manage in the salon include:

- preparing the work area for the next client
- cleaning up the work area before the next client is due
- following instructions from senior members of staff and making sure you carry them out in time
- arriving for work on time.

Time management is also important in your personal life as this can affect how punctual you are at work. Things that you need to time-manage outside of work include:

- job tasks
- homework
- jobs around the house
- time for friends
- time for relaxing.

Time management should work for you and should have some flexibility so that you can alter or change your priorities if you need to.

 Top tip

As an assistant, you should aim to be hard-working and reliable. This means that you work to the best of your abilities and don't need constant supervision. Flexibility is also a great advantage. Try to **adapt** to changing circumstances and situations without complaining.

Develop yourself within your job role (4)

Continuous professional development (CPD)

It is not enough to gain a qualification, as techniques, products and skills are changing and improving all the time, especially with the introduction of new things. Therefore, you must continually try to improve by going on training courses, attending exhibitions, reading **trade journals** and sharing ideas and tips with other therapists.

After you have qualified

Spend every possible moment developing your knowledge and practising your skills. Don't relax just because you have a qualification. Read every book, magazine and trade journal you can lay your hands on to get the latest word on the street.

Attend trade shows, exhibitions and workshops for professional development. Never think you know it all just because you have qualified.

Join professional organisations to keep you informed about new developments and in contact with other therapists that you can share knowledge, advice and good practice with.

Trade journals

The trade journals listed below are written especially for everyone involved in the health and beauty industry and are a good source of professional information. The journals are essential reading for keeping up to date with treatment techniques, new products, cosmetic trends, trade events and celebrity personalities influencing the trade. Journals include:

- *Guild News*
- *Health and Beauty Salon*
- *International Therapist*
- *Professional Beauty*
- *Professional Nails*
- *Salon Today*
- *Tanning World*
- *Today's Therapist.*
- *Hairdressers Journal*
- *The Hairdresser*

Top tip ✓

Visit the Salon International and Professional websites to find about these exhibitions. You can access the websites by going to www.pearsonhotlinks.co.uk and searching for this title.

Courses

There are also courses that are specially designed to help you to continually develop. Information on these can be found from the Habia website and **trade journals**. You can also find out more by visiting the VTCT, Edexcel, and City & Guilds websites. The Connexions Direct and Directgov Careers advice websites may also be useful. You can access these websites by going to www.pearsonhotlinks.co.uk and searching for this title.

National Occupational Standards

These are the standards that describe competent performances necessary for work. The National Occupational Standards are industry-led. This means that the standards are achieved by consultations with:

- salon owners
- industry associations
- practising beauty therapists and hairdressers.

The National Occupational Standards are updated every few years so that they stay current. As new techniques, equipment and treatments develop and become accepted, new standards are developed.

 Top tip

The National Occupational Standards help hair and beauty professionals to keep up to date with new skills and emerging trends. This in turn helps professionals to identify their future development and training needs.

Hair and Beauty Industry Authority (Habia)

Habia is the National Occupational Standards setting body for the hair and beauty industry. Visit the Habia website for lots of information about the hair and beauty industry.

? Memory jogger

1 What does CPD stand for?
2 What does Habia stand for?
3 What are National Occupational Standards?
4 Why is it important to manage your time at work and in your personal life?

Getting ready for assessment

Evidence requirements

You will be observed by your assessor on at least three occasions, two of which will cover your interaction with clients and one of which will cover your interaction with colleagues.

What you cover during your practical assessments

Ranges

From the range you must show that you have:

- participated in all the types of learning opportunity listed.

Performance criteria

In order to perform this unit successfully you must:

- develop effective working relationships with clients and colleagues
- develop yourself within your job role
- identify opportunities to learn.

What you must know

In order to pass this unit you will need to gather evidence to support a consistent performance with colleagues and clients. Assessor observation alone is not enough. You should also collect evidence to show that you have taken part in self-development activities over a period of time. This evidence will also be signed off in your candidate handbook, which you will be given by your assessor. This will be an official record to show that you have covered what you need to.

Get ahead

Complete the table below by matching the qualities to the definitions.

Qualities

Committed to the industry	Reliable
Conscientious	Responsible
Co-operative	Self-motivated
Dedicated	Tolerant
Flexible	Well-presented

Quality needed	Definition of the quality
	Always arriving in good time for work and not taking time off unnecessarily
	Able to adapt to different situations and circumstances without complaining
	Helpful and supportive to others; taking responsibility and making a positive contribution to the team effort
	Accepting that there is room for different views and opinions; never taking offence
	Always looking the part; projecting a professional image
	Working to high standards and being thorough
	Working safely and effectively even when unsupervised, as well as realising the importance of supervision when required
	Showing commitment to the job; being flexible and prepared to put in extra time when necessary
	Able to work well alone without needing others to organise or instruct
	Wanting to succeed as a therapist and prepared to improve standards through continuing professional development whenever the opportunity arises

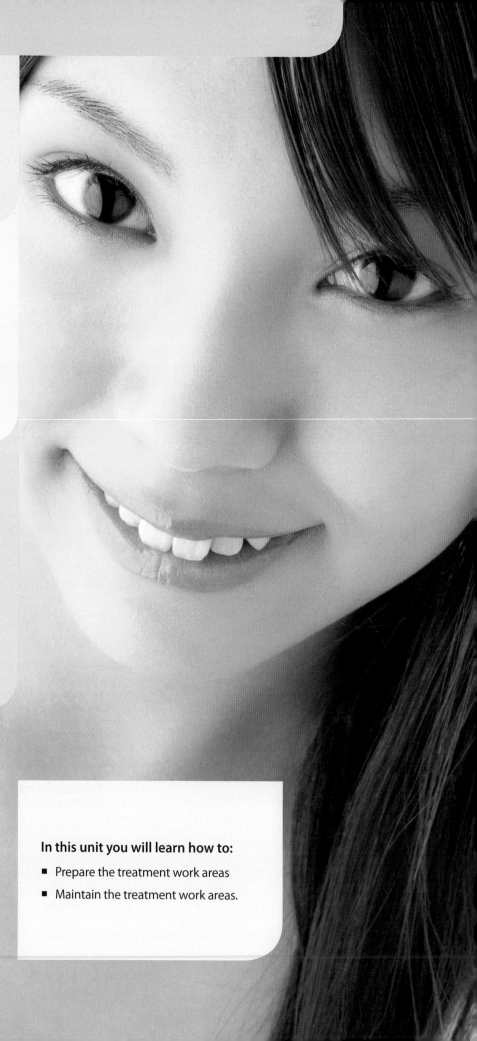

UNIT B1

Prepare and maintain salon treatment work areas

Every beauty treatment and service needs a work area that is clean, tidy, hygienic and inviting. This unit is about preparing and maintaining the work area for waxing, make-up, nail, facial and eye treatments. Setting up involves preparing the tools, equipment and materials needed to carry out the treatment, as well as the seating arrangements for the client and therapist. You will also learn about the disposal of waste after treatments, client records and the importance of your personal hygiene and appearance.

In this unit you will learn how to:

- Prepare the treatment work areas
- Maintain the treatment work areas.

Here are some key terms you may meet in this unit:

Disposal –
throwing away, removal

Incinerated –
disposed of by burning

Thermostatically controlled heating –
heating that is kept at a controlled temperature

Décor –
furnishings and decoration

Ventilation –
circulating fresh air

Magnifying lamp –
a lamp used in treatments that increases the size of something to make it easier to see

Disposables –
things that are meant to be thrown away after they have been used once

Flues –
outlets for fresh air

Dimmer switch –
a light switch that can be turned up or down depending on the level of lighting you want

Extractor fan –
an electric fan often set into a window and used to remove steam, fumes or stale air from a room

Equipped –
set up with the appropriate tools and equipment

Record card –
card where you write important information about the client and their treatments

Prepare the treatment work areas (1)

One of your main duties in the salon will be to assist more senior therapists by setting up the correct materials and equipment needed for a particular treatment or service and by preparing the client.

You will need to know what products, tools and equipment are needed for each of the treatments in the range, and also be able to use a client's **record card** to select materials that will be suitable for that particular client. You will also need to think very carefully about everything that you have learned about health and safety in Unit G20. Make sure your own actions reduce risks to health and safety and put it into practice.

Record cards

A client's record card is a professional record of treatments or services that the client has already had at your salon and is where a therapist can record comments or suggestions for future treatments. Part of your preparation for a treatment will involve obtaining a client's record card from reception. You will need the card to find out what treatment the client is booked in for, so that you know what you need to set up. The client's record card may also give you more information about the client's likes and dislikes, skin type, previous products used and the therapist's methods that will be helpful to you in deciding which products to select.

When you collect a record card for a client from reception, make sure that you check the client's first name, surname and address carefully to make sure you have the correct card. Make sure that you collect the correct record card for the client, as some may share a surname or even a first name.

You will need to hand over the client's record card to the therapist before she starts the treatment.

 Salon life

Jodie was looking for Mrs Jarvis's record card for the therapist, Shruti, but couldn't find it anywhere in the filing box. After five minutes she began to panic – Shruti was really strict about not starting a treatment until everything was ready, and Jodie knew that she would get into trouble if the treatment started late. Eventually the receptionist looked up from her magazine and asked Jodie what the problem was, and when Jodie explained, the receptionist told her to look under Mrs Jarvis's first name, Jan, because that's where she filed it last week. Luckily enough, there it was.

How could this problem be prevented from happening in the future?

What is the best system to use when filing record cards?

The treatment room

As the treatment room is used for a variety of different treatments, it is important that it can be adapted to meet the needs of a range of treatments and is well **equipped**.

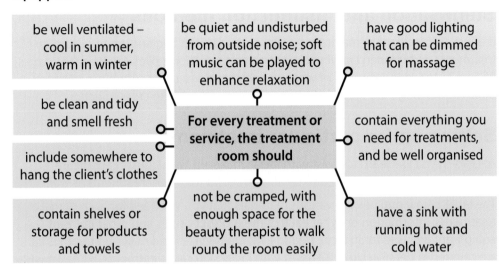

What a good treatment room should be like

You will need to bear all this in mind when preparing the treatment room.

Setting up for treatments

You need to organise the work area so that everything is hygienic and within reach and the trolley is set up with the necessary tools, equipment and products, as well as enough cotton wool and tissues. Your supervisor will show and advise you how to do this until you are able to set up on your own.

Setting up the workspace for any treatment: a checklist

1. The client's **record card** and a pen should be on the trolley ready for the consultation.
2. The gown the client will wear during the treatment should be ready, and there should be a coat hanger or hook available for the client's clothes.
3. Clean towels should be laid out nearby, either on a stool or at the end of the couch.
4. The treatment couch should be prepared with a fitted bottom sheet and a disposable couch roll.
5. The trolley tops and work surfaces should be disinfected and covered with fresh couch roll.
6. The products to be used during the treatment should be laid out on the trolley top.
7. The tools to be used during the treatment should be sterilised and then placed on the trolley top in a jar filled with antiseptic.
8. There should be enough cotton wool and tissues on the trolley to complete the whole treatment.

Prepare the treatment work areas (2)

Sterilisation and disinfection methods

It is just as important to maintain excellent standards of hygiene when setting up for treatments as it is when carrying out the treatments themselves. Look back at pages 26 and 27 to remind yourself of what you need to do to make sure the workspace doesn't encourage the spread of bacteria that could result in cross-infection.

Setting up for particular treatments

At Level 1, you will learn to assist with facial, make-up, manicure and pedicure treatments. However, you need to be able to set up for other treatments as well.

The table below outlines the various materials that you will need for each of these treatments. Information on what each of the products, tools and other items of equipment are used for in facial treatments, nail services and make-up treatments are covered in detail in Units B2 Assist with facial skin care treatments, B3 Assist with day make-up and N1 Assist with nail services.

Treatment	Equipment, tools and products needed
Waxing	Couch, wax station with tools, equipment and materials, protective plastic couch sheet, paper couch roll, client clothing protection, pedal waste bin, tweezers, disinfectant solution in a jar, talcum powder, cotton wool, tissues, skin-cleanser or pre-wax, medium-sized towels, small scissors, selection of different-sized wax strips, wax, after-wax lotion or oil, hand mirror, apron, disposable surgical gloves, pedal bin, clinical waste bin, client **record card** and pen, aftercare leaflet
Eye treatments	Couch, stool, trolley, tools, products, equipment and materials laid out, towels, tissues, orange wood sticks, head band, antiseptic cleansing solution, soothing lotion, hand mirror, damp cotton wool, dry cotton wool, scissors, tweezers, **magnifying lamp**, disposable surgical gloves, tissues, disposable spatula, steel pencil sharpener, eyebrow pencil, disinfectant solution, client record card and pen, pedal bin, disinfectant solution in a jar
Make-up	Couch or beauty chair, trolley, head band, tissues, couch roll, towels, hair clips, cleanser, toner and moisturiser, eye make-up remover, magnifying lamp, bowls, eye make-up, cheek make-up, lip make-up, foundation, powder, concealer, make-up brushes, good lighting, disposable make-up applicators, cosmetic sponges, make-up palette, pencil sharpener, spatulas, orange wood sticks, dry cotton wool, damp cotton wool, hand mirror, artificial eyelashes, client record card and pen
Facial	Couch, stool, trolley, facial tools, products, equipment and materials laid out, towels and **disposables** such as cotton wool, tissues, spatulas, orange wood sticks, pedal bin, disinfectant solution in a jar, head band, gown, mirror, cleansers, toners, moisturisers, massage cream or oil, exfoliants, steamer, selection of different-sized bowls, comedone extractor, mask ingredients to mix or ready prepared masks, mask application brush, magnifying lamp, client record card and pen

Treatment	Equipment, tools and products needed
Manicure	Manicure station, manicure tools, bowls, finger soaking bowl, equipment and materials laid out, towels and **disposables** such as cotton wool, tissues, spatulas, emery boards and orange wood sticks, hand cream, base coat, nail polishes, top coat, cuticle knife, hoof stick, cuticle nippers, nail scissors, buffer, buffing paste, cuticle remover, cuticle massage oil or cream, hand sanitising spray, disinfectant, nail polish remover, nail polish dryer, client **record card** and pen, pedal bin, disinfectant solution in a jar
Pedicure	Pedicure station, pedicure tools, products, equipment and materials laid out, towels and disposables such as cotton wool, tissues, spatulas, emery boards and orange wood sticks, massage cream or foot lotion, base coat, nail polishes, top coat, cuticle knife, hoof stick, cuticle nippers, nail scissors, buffer, buffing paste, cuticle remover, cuticle massage oil or cream, hand sanitising spray, disinfectant, foot file, nail polish remover, nail polish dryer, client record card and pen, pedal bin, disinfectant solution in a jar
Nail art	Manicure station, medium-sized towels, couch roll, dry cotton wool, tissues, hand sanitising spray, emery boards, orange wood sticks, marbling tool, dotting tool, selection of nail art designs, top coat or sealant, nail polishes, nail scissors, nail polish remover, nail polish solvent, water-based and acrylic nail paints, glitter, transfers, foil strips, striping tape, jewellery, gems and rhinestones, client record card and pen
Nail enhancements	Nail workstation, seating, lamp, pedal bin, plastic glasses and safety mask for the nail technician, lint free pads, tissues, nail preparation products, cotton wool discs, cotton buds, orange wood sticks, cuticle knife, cuticle nippers, glass bowl, plastic bowls, dappen dish, scissors, tip cutters, coarse grit file, medium grit file, fine grit file, buffing file, four-sided buffer, medium-sized towels, disinfectant solution in a jar, hand sanitising spray, nail steriliser, acetone, non-acetone polish remover, cuticle oil, client record card and pen

 Get ahead

Find out the tools, equipment and products needed to set up for three more treatments such as massage, Indian head massage and spray tanning and write some key cards for these. Then ask a therapist if you could practise setting up for these during your work experience.

 Top tip

It is helpful to have a checklist of all the tools, products and face/nail basics on a record card that you can keep nearby for reference. Cover the list with a plastic cover so that it doesn't get marked, or have it laminated so that you can wipe it clean.

Prepare the treatment work areas (3)

Environmental conditions

It is important that the environmental conditions in the treatment room are suitable for the client and the treatment. A comfortable treatment area will help to make sure that a salon visit is enjoyable for the client and a satisfying work environment for the therapist.

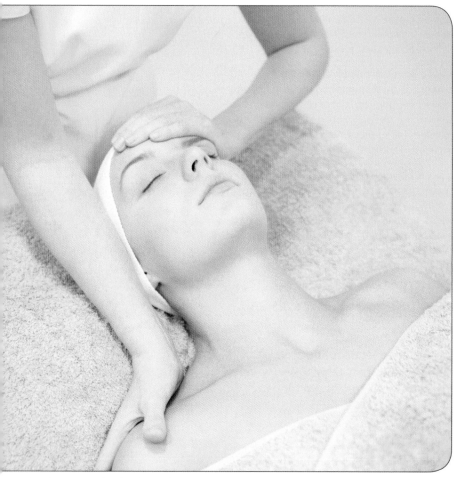

It is important that both the therapist and the client are comfortable

Lighting

Lighting gives a salon atmosphere, so it can have a powerful effect on how the client feels when she walks into the reception, her level of relaxation once in the treatment room, and whether she feels as though she has had a satisfying treatment at the end.

The lighting in a treatment room will depend on the treatment. For example, for make-up the lighting should be bright and not cast shadows, but for facial treatments the light should be relaxing and soft with a **magnifying lamp** available for close work and skin analysis.

The lighting should in any case be:

- bright enough to carry out treatments
- soft enough to enable clients to relax.

Therefore, it is recommended that a treatment room has a good overhead light on a **dimmer switch**, and a magnifying lamp for close work such as skin inspection.

Make sure that:

- you can always see clearly
- you and your client don't squint because lighting is poor, or become dazzled by lights that are too bright
- you always report flickering or faulty lights to your supervisor.

Heating

Clients tend to relax when they have treatments, and therefore their body temperature can drop, so it is important that the salon is warm but not so hot and stuffy that it is uncomfortable or encourages germs to multiply.

A comfortable temperature for beauty therapy work is between 20 and 24°C, with the level of moisture in the air between 40 and 60 per cent. It is also important that the salon is warm enough for clients to undress for treatments.

There are many different heating methods, but some are either too expensive to run on a regular basis or are not good at heating large areas. Therefore, the best method of heating is **thermostatically controlled heating**. This can easily be turned up or down, and every room is fitted with a radiator. When it is installed by a qualified engineer and checked annually, it is the best and most cost effective way to heat a salon.

Ventilation

Circulation of fresh air is needed to make sure that clients and staff don't become drowsy and lacking in energy as well as making sure that people are not made uncomfortable by fumes from products. Fresh air may be gained from open doors and windows, and by having an air-conditioning system in the salon.

In salons and spas that have steam and sauna areas, it is important that the air does not become too damp and humid, so good **ventilation** is essential.

If there is a lack of fresh air:

- illnesses spread because of germs and bacteria circulating around the salon
- a smelly and stuffy atmosphere is created, which is unpleasant for staff and clients
- there is a build-up of fumes from glues, varnish and cleaning products, which can cause headaches and sickness.

Methods of ventilation include **extractor fans**, windows, air vents, doors and **flues**.

General comfort

The general comfort of the client includes making sure that:

- she is seated comfortably
- she is warm
- she is happy with her surroundings
- the noise levels are not too high
- there is relaxing music playing in the background
- there are nice smells
- the **décor** is pleasant and welcoming
- the staff are polite, respectful and professional.

▶▶ Get up and go!

Design a salon based on what you would like to see when you visit one. Think about the lighting, décor, seating and layout. Use swatches of material and colour to decorate it.

? Memory jogger

1 What is thermostatically controlled heating?
2 What can happen if there is no circulation of fresh air in the salon?
3 List five items that you would need to set up for a waxing treatment.
4 List five items that you would need to set up for a pedicure treatment.

Prepare the treatment work areas (4)

Setting up

These are the treatments that you will be involved in setting up for at Level 1.

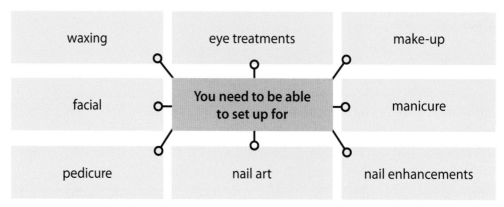

Treatments you need to be able to set up for

As part of your assessment, you will be required to demonstrate that you are able to set up for all of these treatments.

Preparing a client for treatment

Introductions

When the client is brought through to you, or you go to collect her from reception, make sure that you have an open, confident expression. Smile and make eye contact. Greet the client by her name, then introduce yourself and explain that you will be preparing her for her treatment. Ask the client to follow you through to the treatment room. Before the treatment begins, make polite conversation to build a good relationship and help the client to feel at ease.

Polite conversation is:

- asking if she has visited the salon before
- asking if she has regular treatments
- enquiring about other treatments the client has had in the past
- enquiring whether this treatment is for a special occasion
- asking questions about the client's holidays or family
- discussing the weather or light news topics.

Polite conversation is not:

- ignoring the client in order to talk to other members of staff
- talking about yourself or another person, and not asking the client about herself
- moaning about your last client or your job
- telling the client your life story and about your problems at home
- discussing serious news topics, religion or politics.

Client care

Remove and hang up the client's coat, then show her to her seat. Make sure that she is comfortable and provide help where necessary.

Client protection

Protect the client's clothes with a towel or gown.

- For manicure: be especially careful that she is protected from varnish or other products that might stain her clothes. For protection, roll up the client's sleeves to the elbow and then tuck tissue around them.
- For make-up: protect the client's clothing with a make-up cape and protect her hair with a head band.
- For facial treatments: protect the client's upper clothing with a towel and couch roll.

Just before you start

Ask the client to remove her jewellery and show her the bowl in which you will be placing it. Point out that, if she prefers, the client (not you) could put the jewellery in her handbag.

Cleaning your hands

Explain to the client that you are going to wash your hands as this gives her confidence in your cleanliness. Make sure that you dry your hands thoroughly, because wet hands are not clean hands.

Personal presentation and behaviour

Remember that it is important to demonstrate a professional approach to all aspects of the client's visit. Your own personal presentation and behaviour are very important at all times. Looking smart and wearing appropriate protective clothing, such as a salon uniform, will give the client confidence in you. As beauty therapists are on their feet a lot and work very closely with clients, making sure that you maintain good standards of personal hygiene will mean that the client's comfort will not be affected by any body odour. You can find out more about the importance of personal presentation and behaviour on pages 30 and 31.

Appearance: a checklist

Wear smart clothes or uniform – they should be freshly laundered and not smell of smoke or strong perfume.

1 Your uniform or clothes should not be too short or too tight, and must allow for easy movement while carrying out treatments.
2 Your hair should be clean and neat.
3 Wear light, but attractive, day make-up – definitely not heavy make-up.
4 Your nails should be neatly manicured – no chipped nail varnish.
5 Keep your breath fresh – no tobacco smells.
6 If you wear jewellery, it should be simple and kept to a minimum.

? Memory jogger

1 Give two examples of polite conversation and two examples of impolite conversation.

2 Circulation of fresh air is needed to make sure that clients and staff don't become:

A Drowsy and lacking in energy

B Loud and talkative

C Relaxed and chilled

D Grumpy and irritated

3 Why should you tell your clients that you are going to wash your hands?

Maintain the treatment work areas (1)

It is not enough to prepare a perfect work area. It is also your responsibility to keep it clean, hygienic and looking professional at all times. To do this you must tidy up as you go along, ensure waste **disposal** is safe and, after the treatment, make sure that the area is left in a state that is suitable for the next treatment (remembering of course that it may be a different therapist and different client that could be using it next).

Safe disposal of waste

As soon as you have used cotton wool, tissues or other **disposables** you must put them in a foot pedal bin immediately. Any other type of bin is unsuitable as you will have to touch the lid to open the bin and that means your hands will not be clean and you could risk cross-infection.

For treatments such as waxing where there may be skin fluids such as blood, the waste must be disposed of in a clinical waste bin. The waste in this bin is collected by the local council and **incinerated**.

Top tips

- Tidy up as you go – it will save time later.
- Replace bottle tops straight away.
- Place waste in the bin straight away. This is also good practice with regard to health and safety because:
  - nail varnish gives off very strong fumes
  - used cotton wool and tissues contain germs.
- During manicures and pedicures, use the nail varnish drying time to clear things away such as dirty towels and water in the manicure bowl. Clean tools and place them back in the steriliser.
- During facials, use the time when the mask is on to tidy away small items and get fresh warm water. However, you must do this very quietly so as not to disturb the client.
- If you are allowed to watch as your senior therapist is carrying out other treatments, keep an eye out for:
  - bits on the floor that may need to be put in the bin or swept up
  - tools and equipment that may need washing or disinfection
  - bottle tops that may need replacing.

Checking and cleaning equipment

The life of the equipment used depends on thorough and safe cleaning methods that follow the manufacturer's instructions. Each piece of equipment when new comes with instructions on how to clean and maintain it so that it lasts a long time. You will not be responsible for the cleaning and maintenance of equipment without supervision. However, it is your responsibility to report any possible problems that you may see with the equipment such as:

- trailing wires
- faulty plugs
- dirty machines and attachments
- broken parts.

All equipment should be checked annually by a qualified electrician. After it has been checked it will have a green safety sticker put on it which tells people that it is safe to use and has been checked. The sticker also has the date that it was tested on and when the next test is due.

 Get up and go!

Find out when the equipment in your salon was last tested by a qualified electrician.

Leaving work areas clean and hygienic

When the client has left the treatment area, the following things need to be done:

- all bedding and towels washed
- products tidied away
- worktops and trolleys disinfected
- tools sterilised
- **disposables** thrown away
- equipment cleaned
- new bedding or couch roll laid out.

The exact way that things are done depends on the salon's own methods, so you will need to find out what your supervisor expects and what other things they would expect to be carried out so that the room is left in a state that is fit for the next treatment.

When you have finished the treatment, make sure that you leave the workspace perfect. It may help if you take a mental photograph of the area before you set up, which means trying to remember where and how everything was before you started and then put it back exactly how it was.

 Top tip

Remember to allow a small amount of time between treatments to tidy and clean the treatment area, so that it is ready for the next client. It is bad practice for a client to enter a room or cubicle that is either unprepared or is a mess of dirty towels and has products from the last treatment spread all over the trolley.

Maintain the treatment work areas (2)

Daily and weekly cleaning

In addition to clearing and preparing the work area after a treatment, the salon furnishings and equipment should be kept clean at all times. The best way to make sure that everything is cleaned regularly is to write a list of all the cleaning jobs that need doing. There will be some jobs that need doing every day and others that are required only once a week. If a salon has an 'end-of-day' and a 'weekly' cleaning list, these jobs can be ticked off and signed each time they are done. The salon supervisor and employees can then easily check to see what cleaning jobs still need doing. The table below is an example of a daily cleaning list for a treatment room.

Daily cleaning job	Date and therapist's signature				
	23/11	24/11	25/11	26/11	27/11
Clean wax pot	SJ				
Sweep floor	SJ				
Wipe down work surfaces and trolleys	JD				
Change couch roll on trolleys	LL				
Sanitise, sterilise and put away tools	LL				
Clear away all equipment	LL				
Lay out fresh towels	JD				
Clean mirrors	SJ				

» Get up and go!

Think about the salon where you are learning or carrying out your work experience. Create a table with two columns: end-of-day cleaning and weekly cleaning. Write down as many cleaning jobs as you can think of.

When you have finished, compare your list with those of other learners in the class.

Storage of records, materials and equipment

Client records

These must be stored in line with the Data Protection Act 1998. This legislation is designed to protect client privacy and confidentiality, so all client records must be stored in a secure way such as in a lockable filing cabinet or, if stored electronically on a computer, this must be password protected.

If you are given the responsibility to put away client records, you must treat them confidentially and not show anyone the information. You must also follow the salon guidelines for storing these.

Tools and equipment

Each salon will have its own methods of safe storage of tools and equipment. However, the most important thing that you can help with is to make sure that all of these are cleaned, disinfected and sterilised before they are put away to avoid cross-contamination.

Sharp tools should always be stored so that they cannot be knocked off a shelf as they could land on someone's feet. They should also never be stored in uniform pockets.

Electrical equipment must always be turned off and unplugged when not in use and the electrical leads must not be left trailing on the floor. An important thing to remember when storing **magnifying lamps** is that they should never be left in sunlight, as this could cause a reflection that may result in a fire.

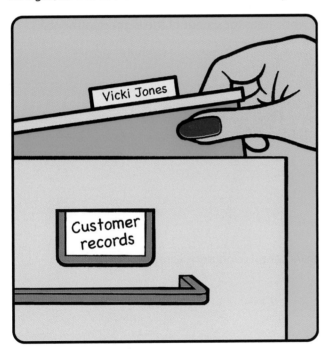

Clients' record cards must be stored securely

? Memory jogger

1 Under what act should client records be stored?
2 List five things that you would need to do at the end of a treatment.
3 What is the most hygienic bin to use in a salon treatment area for general treatment waste?
4 Why should you follow manufacturer's instructions?

Get ahead

When an electrical appliance is checked by an electrician and a green sticker placed on it showing that it is safe to be used, what is this process called?

Getting ready for assessment

Evidence requirements

You will be observed by your assessor on at least three occasions and must demonstrate in your everyday work that you have met the standards for preparation and maintenance of the beauty therapy work area.

What you must cover during your practical assessments

Ranges

In your candidate handbook you will have a list of ranges that you must cover during your assessment.

In this unit you must have covered the ranges below:

1 Prepared and maintained work areas for six out of the eight treatments below:

- waxing
- eye treatments
- make-up
- facial
- manicure
- pedicure
- nail art
- nail enhancements.

2 Prepared all types of environmental conditions listed below:

- lighting
- heating
- **ventilation**
- general comfort.

It is good practice to cover as many ranges as possible during each assessment. This will prevent you from having to take too many additional assessments because there are many ranges that you have not managed to cover.

Performance criteria

You must demonstrate during a practical observation by your tutor that you have:

- prepared for the treatments safely and hygienically
- considered the previous client records for further information on the set-up
- made sure that all equipment and tools have been cleaned and sterilised

- made sure that your appearance, hygiene and protection have been demonstrated
- given the correct client record to the therapist
- disposed of waste in the correct way
- checked and cleaned the equipment following the manufacturer's instructions
- cleared away and stored everything in the correct way after the treatment
- left the work area in a fit state for the next treatment.

Throughout your observations you will also need to make sure that you pay attention to health, safety and hygiene throughout, as well as presenting yourself well, so read through Unit G20 Make sure your own actions reduce risks to health and safety before any practical assessment just to refresh your memory.

Carrying out a practical treatment using unhygienic tools or without carrying out a risk assessment of your work area to avoid accidents happening will mean that you are not safe to do a treatment and therefore could mean that you do not pass your assessment or, perhaps worse, are stopped from doing your assessment.

What you must know

In order to pass this unit, you will need to gather evidence during the teaching and learning of this unit before your assessor observes your practical performance. You will gather this during class work and further study and will probably file it in a portfolio of evidence. This evidence will also be signed off in your candidate handbook which you will be given by your assessor. This will be an official record to show that you have covered what you need to.

 Top tips

- There is such a lot to remember when setting up for a treatment or service. Have key cards for each treatment and service that list all of the tools, products and materials required. Small record cards or postcards are a suitable size for this.
- If you are unsure about anything it is very important that you ask your supervising therapist – don't be worried about asking questions.

 Salon life

Mary and Samira started work at La Belle at the same time. They were both at school most of the week and spent one day a week at the salon. It was a very busy salon and there was always so much to do to help the senior therapists. Mary loved the work but felt that she ended up doing most of the clearing up and Samira got the better job of preparing the rooms. Not only that, because Samira did the setting-up the senior therapists praised her all the time because they loved the organised, fresh-smelling rooms that they took their clients into. Unfortunately they didn't notice Mary: by the time she had cleaned out the rooms, collected the laundry and emptied the bins it was time for Samira to do her bit, lighting candles, preparing cotton wool and tissues and changing the music. It all just seemed a little unfair, but Mary didn't want to make a fuss. Mary had asked Samira if they could share the different jobs, but Samira had a way with words and said that Mary had the most important role.

Do you think that this would be a fair share of duties in the salon? If not, why?

How would you deal with this situation if it happened to you?

UNIT G2

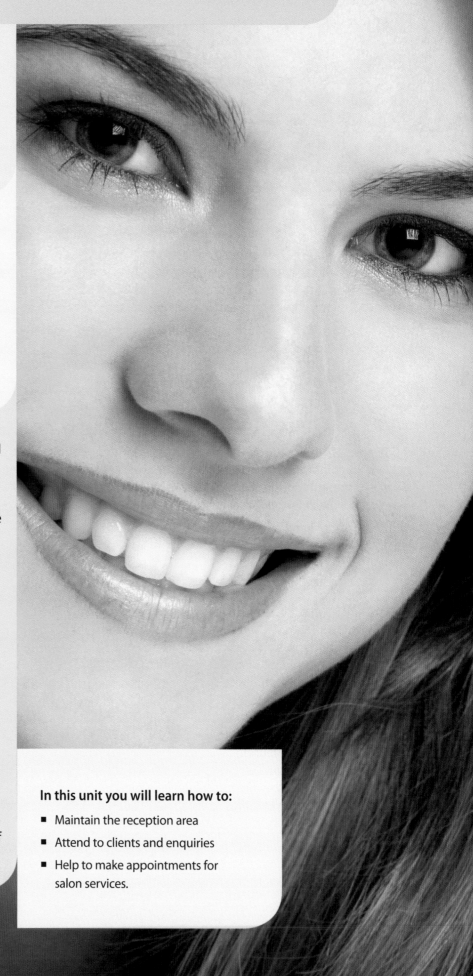

Assist with salon reception duties

Although some salons employ an experienced receptionist who is not a beauty therapist, it is more usual for existing beauty staff to take turns in running reception. Assisting with salon reception duties will involve keeping the reception clean, tidy and organised, making appointments, attending to clients, selling products and handling money. You will be able to use your knowledge of treatments and products to give clients good advice, and assisting with reception will also help you to improve your understanding of the working pressures that therapists experience.

Many clients will decide whether or not they like a salon within moments of arriving in the reception area, so you need to make sure that the client's first and lasting impression is a good one. Communication skills are very important, and you need to be enthusiastic, cheerful, helpful, professional and respectful to every client. By doing a good job with assisting with reception, you will contribute to the successful running and good reputation of your salon.

In this unit you will learn how to:

- Maintain the reception area
- Attend to clients and enquiries
- Help to make appointments for salon services.

Here are some key terms you may meet in this unit:

Professional – high standards and a good attitude

Respectful – treating others with politeness and thought

Discreet – careful in your choice of words, loudness of speech and able to act in a confidential manner

Confidential – keeping things private

Slang – informal language and speech

Potential clients – people who are interested in beauty treatments and may use the salon in the future

Authority – the limits of your power and what you are allowed to do

Confidentiality – keeping all personal information that a client tells you private

Stock rotation – bringing the older stock items to the front of the display or for use and placing the new ones at the back

Shelf life – the life of the product before it passes its sell-by date

Formal – speaking or acting respectfully in a way that is not familiar to someone

Complementary therapies – treatments such as reflexology aromatherapy and Indian head massage that were originally from different cultures or countries

Maintain the reception area (1)

Remember that the reception area is the first point of contact for clients. Although the booking of appointments, both on the telephone and in person, is obviously a key purpose of a reception area, there are many other reasons why a beauty salon needs a reception.

- It is where information and help on treatments and products are provided.
- It is where the sale of products and the handling of money for product sales and treatments take place.
- It is used for handing out brochures and price lists to **potential clients**.
- Window and cabinet display for products, and possibly even flower displays, will be set up here.
- It is where clients are looked after, both before and after treatment.

Maintaining the reception area will involve attention to all these things.

The reception area from outside

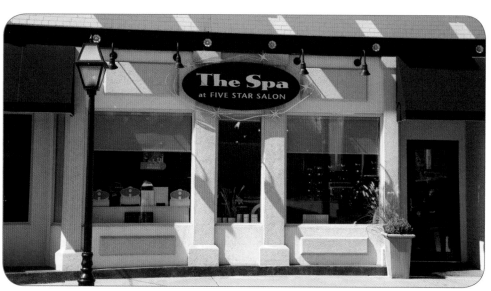

The outside of the beauty salon should encourage people to enter

For people in the street – who may be potential clients – the reception area is an extension of the shop window. As they look into the salon, they will see the reception area. It is therefore important that this area appears organised and very clean, and gives a good impression of the salon.

The shop front should encourage clients to enter, so ideally it will have:

- plants or hanging baskets
- information about the salon's hours of opening
- signs saying what treatments are available
- clean windows
- a freshly painted exterior – not cracked or peeling
- a well-swept front.

Get ahead ⬆

Design your own reception area. Think about what you need and where everything should be placed. Design it by creating a virtual reception either on the computer or by making a model using swatches of material and colour schemes.

However, although it is good to have a central position in a busy shopping area for a beauty salon, it is best not to be in full view of passing people. Blinds can therefore be used to screen waiting clients from public view and to shade display products from the hot sun.

Inside the reception area

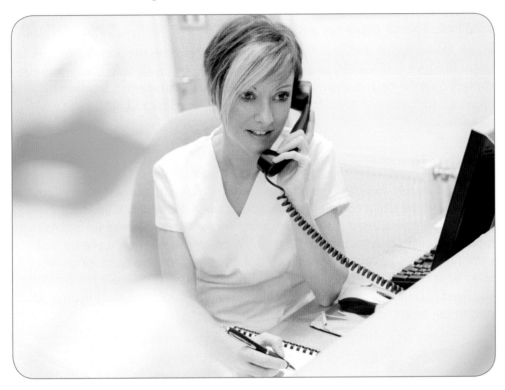

The salon reception desk should be neat and tidy at all times

When a client enters the reception area, he or she needs to feel welcome and at ease with the staff and surroundings. It is also important that clients have the impression that the salon is being run **professionally** and efficiently.

The whole reception area should be well lit, warm, fresh-smelling and, most importantly, spotless. There should be a comfortable seating area for waiting clients with a selection of up-to-date magazines and promotion leaflets. The temperature should be warm in the cooler seasons and airy in the summer months. Refreshments in the form of tea, coffee and mineral water should be available for clients, both before and after treatment. Soothing background music should be played to create a relaxed atmosphere and enhance clients' experience of the salon.

In the reception area there should be a locked product display cabinet from which clients can view and purchase skin, body and nail care products. All salon staff should be familiar with the products so that they can advise clients. If you notice that stocks are low, inform the correct staff member.

The décor of the salon should reflect the image that the salon wants to achieve. The colours and textures of the walls, ceilings, furniture, linen and towels should work together to create the correct atmosphere of tranquility and relaxation. A more modern and funky approach to design is not recommended as it can date very quickly. It is best to aim for a classic design, using pale colours for a fresh look.

 Get up and go!

What beauty salons are there in your area? Have you visited them? If you have, think about their reception area, what they do right and what they could improve on. Discuss in pairs or as a group.

Maintain the reception area (2)

Stationery and paperwork

The reception desk should be positioned so that the receptionist can greet everyone that enters the salon. It should be neat and tidy at all times with just the essentials on view – the cash till, the appointment book, price lists, appointment cards, the telephone, a pencil, eraser and pen.

Ideally, the reception desk should have shelving underneath the desk. This allows for larger amounts of stationery and paperwork to be stored in an orderly way without cluttering up the desk. It also makes it easy to see at a glance when brochures, appointment cards and appointment sheets are getting low and need to be reordered.

Products

Beauty salons rely on selling products to boost their takings and, although all staff are involved, the sale is completed at reception when the money is taken for the product. The typical items that beauty salons sell are skin care, make-up and nail care products. These are attractive products to clients – we all love new make-up, nail varnishes and skin creams. If attractively displayed and on show to passing clients, it is likely that these products will sell easily. In order to assist in the sale of a product, you need to be familiar with the prices offered in your salon. Information on product pricing can be found on page 83.

Top tip ✓

If you notice that salon stationery is getting low, take responsibility and inform the member of staff who deals with stock and ordering.

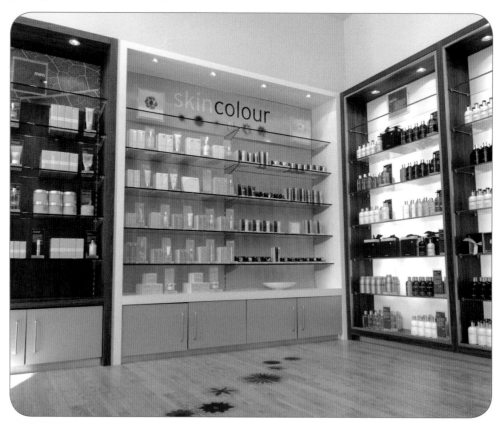

A product display

Product display

The best way to display products is in the reception area in a locked glass-fronted cabinet. The cabinet should be positioned away from the glare and direct heat of the sun. This is because the heat could:

- bleach the boxes
- cause the products to thicken and separate.

The products should be neatly arranged and clearly visible to the eye. There should be enough items on display to catch people's interest without them looking cluttered. One or two of each item that you stock is enough.

The products should look as new as when they were first put on display. It is therefore important that they are taken out and dusted regularly. If the products are dusty or look old, it will discourage people from buying them. Keep an eye out for any damage, loose packaging, cracks and leaks – you will need to remove any breakages or faulty products from the display cabinet and report them straight away to the relevant person.

The stock cupboard

The main stock should be stored out of view, but in an easy-to-reach location, so that when a sale is made the product can be accessed easily. It is also good for the client to see that she is purchasing a new product and not one that has been used for display purposes.

Correct storage of stock

To prevent spoilage and extend a product's **shelf life**, it should generally be kept:

- dry and cool
- in a dark place away from sunlight
- away from naked flames
- in an airtight container – for example, if you open a face cream and then try to reseal it, it will be unfit for sale.

However, you should always check the manufacturer's instructions about correct product storage.

Product shelf life

Remember that all stock has a shelf life. This means that it has a recommended time limit during which it should be stored or used. After this time, the product can go off, making it unfit for use and unsellable to customers. Outward signs that a product has gone off are:

- an unpleasant smell
- separation – this is when a cream or lotion is no longer completely mixed together and becomes part cream, part liquid
- thickness – if a product has passed its sell-by date or has been open to the air, it can turn hard where it becomes dehydrated
- discolouration – this is when a product changes colour.

Maintain the reception area (3)

Products

Stock rotation

To make sure that products are used within their **shelf life** and do not go off, a system known as **stock rotation** is used.

- New stock received from suppliers is placed at the back of the storage area so that it is sold last.
- Stock already on the premises is stored at the front and is sold first.

If your salon does not sell a lot of stock, then products will be sitting in storage for some time and sell-by dates will need to be checked on a regular basis and less stock carried. When stock is reaching its sell-by date, salons usually promote it as a special offer and sell it at a discounted price.

> **» Get up and go!**
>
> Think of a beauty product that you would like to sell. To make sure stock is sold before its sell-by date, you are going to advertise this product at a discounted price and design a 'special offer' poster to be displayed in the reception area. The special offer could be a percentage or a half-price discount, or a buy-one-get-one-free offer.
>
> Remember to make the poster colourful, tasteful and easy to read. It must be eye-catching.

Recording stock levels

Stock should be checked in and out of the salon using either a stock sheet (the manual method) or a computer (a computerised system). If stock levels are not recorded properly, it is impossible to know when to reorder products and which ones to reorder. It is also impossible to check which products are popular with clients and whether any have been stolen.

When stock is counted on a regular basis, this is called a stock take.

Stock taking

When carrying out a stock take, there should be a list of available stock for sale and salon use, either in a file, a stock sheet or on the computer. All staff should record when a new product is opened for use in the salon, and when an old product is empty and the bottle or tub is discarded. They should also keep a record of any sales and breakages. Ideally, a stock take should be done each week so that available stock is counted and a list made of new stock to be ordered. A stock take is best done using a stock sheet.

Using a stock sheet

When new stock arrives in the salon, each individual item needs to be entered into the amount column. It is not advisable to enter the total amount of stock in one cell, as this would make it difficult to count out. For example, if you receive four cleansers, you should mark '1' in the amount column four times. In this way, stock can easily be checked out by crossing through each '1'.

Once you have entered the product and the amount of stock, then you can complete the column for 'Date in'. When stock is removed from the stock cupboard, you should complete the columns for 'Date out' and 'Reason'.

Product	Date in	Amount	Date out	Reason	Signature
Cleanser for dry skin	20/09/10	I I I	28/09/10	sale	SJT
		I I I I I			
		I I			
		I			
Toner for dry skin	20/09/10	I	01/10/10	damaged – reported	LL
		I			

An example of a simple stock sheet

Possible reasons for stock out that you may put on the stock sheet are:

- sale
- display
- salon use
- damaged or broken.

The person who has removed the stock must sign in the 'Signature' column. When more stock that is new arrives, enter it in the space at the bottom of the chart with the date, so it is obvious which entries are new and which are old stock.

» Get up and go!

You have noticed the following problems:

- a damaged product
- low stationery
- there is only one moisturiser for sensitive skin remaining in the cabinet.

Who do you report these problems to?

Using information from your place of work or your training school or college, write out and complete the table below. You may want to add any other things that need reporting.

Problem to report	Member of staff to report to
Low on price lists and appointment cards	
Broken products	
Damaged goods	
Low on make-up and skin care products	

? Memory jogger

1 What is stock rotation?
2 What is shelf life?
3 What is a stock take?
4 What is a product display?

Attend to clients and enquiries (1)

When you are assisting on reception, you are the first point of contact for every person who enters your salon. You are on show to everyone, and so your appearance, attitude and communication skills are very important. Remember that working in the beauty industry involves helping clients to feel relaxed and better about themselves, and so you need to be polite, positive and attentive at all times when attending to the visitors to your salon and listening to their enquiries.

Personal presentation

It is essential that your appearance is of a very high standard. Most clients will think that the way the receptionist appears reflects the standards in the salon. If the staff are sloppy and untidy in appearance, then a client may think that the salon is sloppy and untidy too. Some tips on how to ensure that your appearance is **professional** can be found in Units G20 and G3.

Communication

As a receptionist, you will be greeting clients; booking appointments; answering queries; selling products; dealing with complaints; answering the telephone; taking messages and passing on information, perhaps from a client to a therapist, or from a therapist to a client, or from one member of your team to another. Being able to communicate positively and effectively is essential to your role.

There are different forms of communication:

- Oral – speaking to another person. This includes speaking by telephone or face-to-face conversations.
- Body language – eye contact, nodding or smiling, for example; not spoken language.
- Visual – pictures that communicate information such as adverts, posters, magazines and brochures.
- Written – for example, letters, memos, faxes, text messages and email.

Communicating effectively involves making use of all of these methods and knowing which method to use for a particular situation. Often you will use a combination of methods. Your body language and the way you say things can be just as important as the words you use. In Unit G3 Contribute to the development of effective working relationships you learned about positive and negative communication. Think about some of the examples of negative communication, such as yawning or slouching. If you were feeling tired or worried about a personal issue, you might communicate a negative message to a client without meaning to. You must always maintain a professional attitude.

You must also remember that effective communication is a two-way process. It is about receiving as well as giving information. Its success depends on how clearly we can make ourselves understood as well as how clearly we can understand others. Noting down information, being prompt when passing on messages and using clear language when you speak are all very important, but so too are listening carefully to what other people say and interpreting any other messages that someone might be trying to communicate to you. Do all that you can to make sure that you communicate as clearly as possible.

Top tip

It is very rude and unprofessional to keep a client waiting without keeping her fully informed of what is going on. If a client realises that she will not be dealt with immediately, then she can decide whether to wait in the salon or return later. If a client is not kept informed of this, she may become impatient and unhappy.

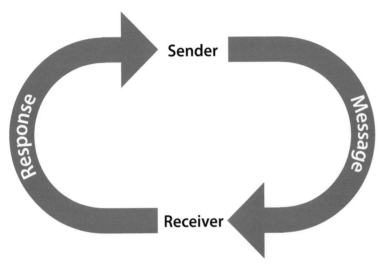

The process of communication

 Get up and go!

Below is a list of some of the different tasks that a receptionist may need to communicate. Think about each task and identify the best method of communication to use for each of them. Some of the methods are quicker than others, so you will need to prioritise. In other words, decide how important or urgent the message is, then decide on the best method of communication.

You may like to copy the table below then draw a line to connect each task with the correct method as they are not in the correct order.

Task	Method of communication
To let a therapist know that her next client has cancelled an appointment	Invoice
To inform all staff of the extended opening times in the salon	Meeting
To let all staff know about the reception duty rota	Memo
To tell customers about new products	Notice board
To inform a client how much she owes	Leaflet
To bill a customer for her course of treatments	Spoken word

Attend to clients and enquiries (2)

Welcoming clients

The value of a warm welcome for clients must not be underestimated – a cheerful and bright smile that is genuine will instantly put a client at ease, whether she has arrived for an appointment or to make an enquiry.

- A **professional** yet welcoming greeting would be: 'Good morning/afternoon Ms/Mrs/Miss/Mr ...' (use the client's name if you know it). 'How can I help?'
- A professional goodbye would be: 'We hope to see you again soon. Goodbye Ms/Mrs/Miss/Mr ...' (while holding the door open for the person).

Welcoming clients: a checklist

1 Make eye contact without staring and keep your facial expressions open – don't frown, roll your eyes or glare.

2 Don't chat to other members of staff while a client is with you, unless it is to answer an enquiry about their appointment or treatment.

3 Vary the tone of your voice so that you don't sound bored and disinterested. Ask helpful questions to show interest in your client.

4 Be caring and **discreet**. Remember, many clients feel quite nervous about visiting a beauty salon.

Taking the client's money

A very important part of being on a reception desk is taking the client's payment for treatment. There are many different methods and it takes a while to be able to carry out the different ways accurately and efficiently, especially if the reception is very busy. You will not be expected to do this alone. A senior colleague or receptionist will instruct and help you to make sure that you can do it properly as it is an extremely responsible job and very easy to make mistakes.

Types of payment

Products or treatment can be paid for with cash, cheques, credit cards, debit cards or gift vouchers.

When taking money it is always a good idea to say to the client how much the product or treatment is, state how much money they give you, and then give the receipt and/or change to the client, stating this amount also.

Confirming appointments

A client who has arrived for an appointment is referred to as an 'existing booking'. When a client arrives for an appointment, take the client's appointment details, confirm them with her and have them checked by a senior staff member. Ask the client to take a seat in the reception area, and offer her magazines and refreshments

Top tip ☑

Concentrate on your numeracy and ICT skills. Numeracy skills are very important for work on a reception. Taking payment, pricing products and working out time needed for appointments all need you to use maths. ICT skills are also important as many tills and client record systems are electronic.

in line with your salon's policy. Then inform the therapist who will be treating her that her next client has arrived.

Client enquiries

To be in a good position to deal with client enquiries, you need to know about the treatments offered in your salon, how long each treatment takes, which therapists can offer them, how much they cost and the benefits they offer, as well as information about the different products that are available for clients to buy. Your supervisor or manager will guide you as you learn how to deal with these sorts of enquiries.

The most common types of treatments and services offered are:

- manicures
- pedicures
- waxing
- facials
- eye treatments such as brow shaping, lash and brow tinting
- body massage
- ear piercing
- nail extensions
- spray tanning.

Some salons also offer **complementary therapies** such as:

- aromatherapy
- reflexology
- hot stone therapy
- Indian head massage.

Prices for services and treatments

Prices of treatments and services vary a great deal across different towns, cities and regions of the UK, so it is important to become familiar with the prices of the treatments offered in the salon that you work in.

Product pricing

As with services, product pricing varies, so again it is important that you are familiar with the prices of the products offered in your salon. Prices are usually set by working out:

- cost price – the price the salon buys the product at
- an additional mark-up that the salon decides in order to make a profit
- these two things will result in a recommended retail price (RRP).

For example:

Nail varnish: Cost price £5.50 + salon mark-up £4.00 = RRP £9.00

> **>> Get up and go!**
>
> Calculate the following:
>
> - A client's bill comes to £58 and she wants to book and pay for a pedicure for her friend next week which costs £30.
> - She wants to pay for her bill using two different methods of payment: a gift voucher for £25 plus the rest on her credit card.
> - How much would she need to pay on her credit card?

Attend to clients and enquiries (3)

Giving information on products and services

Below are some examples of questions that a client might ask about beauty treatments and products.

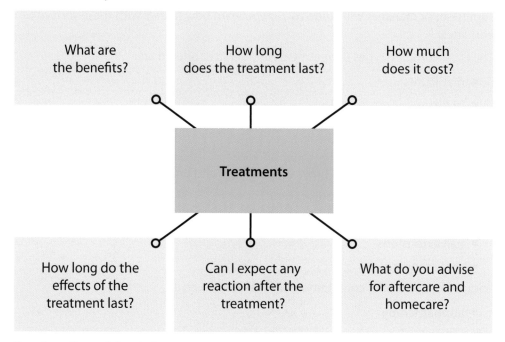

Questions clients might ask about a treatment

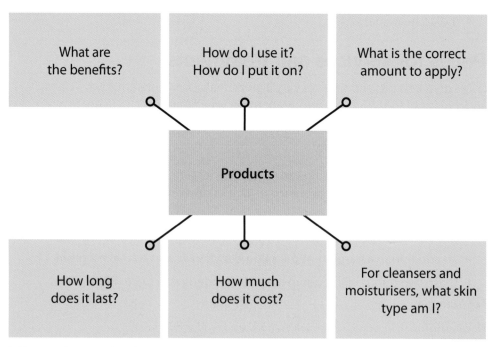

Questions clients might ask about a product

Products for sale

In pairs, choose a product and learn about it for 10–15 minutes.

Now test your knowledge. One of you will be the client, the other will be the therapist. The client asks the therapist questions about the product, for the therapist to answer. When you have finished, swap roles and repeat this activity for a treatment.

How much did you know? Imagine having to give information about all the products and treatments that are available in a beauty salon.

It takes time and practice to be able to advise clients on the different products for sale and the type of treatments available. As a trainee, you can expect to be asked many questions to which you will not know the answer but, with time, the help of your manager and perseverance on your part, you will gradually learn what the best advice to give is.

You may also receive enquiries from suppliers, but you will not have the **authority** to deal with these apart from taking a message to pass on to the appropriate person. It is important to act **professionally** and use good communication techniques when dealing with all visitors and enquiries to the salon.

When dealing with enquiries and requests, it is essential that you keep within the limits of your own authority. There will be many times when you need to pass an enquiry or request on to a senior member of staff. For example, if one of the salon's suppliers needs to speak to the manager but she is at lunch and won't return for ten minutes, you should offer the supplier a coffee, show him or her the list of products that the manager wrote down in the morning, and explain that the manager will confirm what is needed when she returns from lunch.

 Top tip

It is best to refer a client to a senior member of staff rather than give out incorrect information. The consequences of giving a client incorrect information could be a reaction to a product, a returned product, or a client complaint.

? Memory jogger

1 What enquiries might you have on reception?
2 What other skills might be useful while working on reception?
3 List three general beauty treatments that might be booked on reception.
4 List three complementary beauty treatments that might be booked on reception.

Attend to clients and enquiries (4)

Dealing with complaints

When a complaint is made, the reception desk is normally the first point of contact. From there, the complaint will be passed on to the appropriate senior member of staff. As there will probably be clients waiting in reception while someone makes a complaint, it is very important that complaints are dealt with politely and without aggression. It would be embarrassing for waiting clients, and give a very poor impression of the salon, if a complaint was not handled well.

Most people dread having to deal with a complaint. Some people are very good at calming down an angry client or tackling a difficult situation. Other people react in a way that only seems to make the situation worse.

You will not be expected to sort out a complaint until much further into your training. While you are a trainee, you should pass the complaint on to the correct member of staff.

Most complaints can be sorted out quickly and easily because most clients are reasonable and know exactly what will make them happy again. On rare occasions, however, you may experience a more difficult situation that tests your patience. Whatever the situation, the client making the complaint should be gently moved away from the reception area into a quieter area of the salon, where the complaint can be dealt with privately.

Top tips ✓

- Watch and learn from your workmates. You will see good and bad ways of dealing with a complaint.
- A client who complains is giving you a second chance. An unhappy client who doesn't complain will probably tell others how dissatisfied she is and never return.

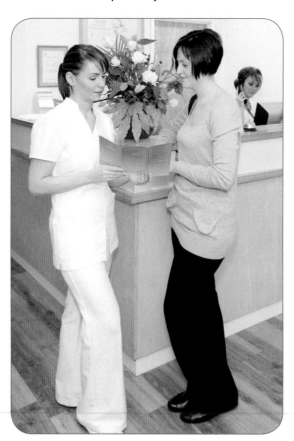

Having a positive influence

When dealing with complaints, there are qualities and skills that will help to solve the problem in the best way. These are:

- patience
- acting on a complaint, not reacting
- listening skills
- deciding on the main facts
- remaining calm
- keeping an open expression
- positive body language.

You can have a positive influence

Don't forget that one of the most important and effective ways to deal with a complaint is to apologise to the client for the fact that she is unhappy with the situation. Your client could be unhappy with:

- how he or she has been treated
- the standard of treatment
- an incorrect appointment
- a faulty product that he or she purchased
- an unpleasant skin reaction to a treatment or product.

An apology will go a long way to helping your client feel better about the situation and the treatment received from the salon.

Answering the telephone

When assisting on reception, you will have to answer the telephone. Remember that answering the telephone at work is not the same as speaking on the phone to friends or family. Take care to pronounce words clearly, using good communication skills, and never use **slang**. Smile! Even though the other person can't see you, you will sound friendlier.

The most acceptable method of telephone greeting is to use a polite greeting first, add the name of the salon, and then ask how you can help. Each salon usually has a preferred method of greeting when answering the telephone, and they will train their staff in this. It is good to be polite and **respectful** without being too **formal**.

Taking messages

You will frequently be asked to take messages during your time on reception. This must be done promptly, accurately and in writing that is neat and easy to read.

Details that you will need to write are:

- the date and time of the message or call
- who the message is from
- who the message is for
- what the message is about
- how important the message is – urgent, important or no immediate hurry
- the caller's name, company name and contact details (telephone number).

It is very important that you remember to write down all this information, because any details that are missed could result in a complete misunderstanding. Don't rely on memory. When the salon is busy and you have lots of other things to remember, it is easy to forget the details of a message.

 Top tip

Message pads can help to jog a person's memory. These list all the information you should write down when taking a message and can be purchased from stationery shops.

 Get up and go!

Design your own message sheet. You may like to do this by hand or on a computer. When you have finished, photocopy the sheet a few times. You may like to use it when you are on reception to see how it works.

Attend to clients and enquiries (5)

Confidentiality

Remember that, as a receptionist, you are in a position of responsibility and there are certain salon and legal requirements that you must meet.

Confidentiality is central to the running of a **professional** beauty salon. A client must feel confident that any personal information she gives remains private and that the staff don't gossip about her behind her back. Gossiping about clients is unprofessional behaviour that breaks a client's trust and is extremely disrespectful to the client.

What information is confidential?

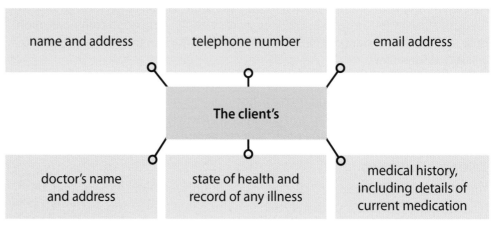

name and address	telephone number	email address

The client's

doctor's name and address	state of health and record of any illness	medical history, including details of current medication

Confidential information

 Top tip

Information is given by a client to a therapist or receptionist in confidence. This information must remain private unless it is illegal or could hurt someone. If you are unsure or worried about confidentiality, always check with your manager.

Record systems

Confidential information, such as client records, should never be visible to other clients or to members of staff not treating the client. They should be stored in lockable drawers underneath the reception desk.

While on reception duty, you will see clients' private records. You have no right to pass these on or to talk about them to anyone, except other members of staff who need to know because they may carry out a treatment on or look after the client. Even then, you must only discuss client details when it concerns a work-related matter and you have the permission of the client. If you are unsure about what to do, ask a senior member of staff.

The Data Protection Act 1998

The Data Protection Act covers many different working practices. The section that is important to beauty therapists is the one that describes the correct privacy methods that should be in place in a salon. These privacy methods ensure that it is difficult for other people to get hold of, look at or use a person's private details without permission, for any reason.

The act states that beauty therapists should treat a client's personal details in confidence – that means keeping it private. It is against the law to give out someone's personal information without his or her permission.

 Top tips

- Never leave a record card on the reception desk in full view of everyone.
- Never allow clients to view a person's private records on a computer screen.

>> **Get up and go!**

Use the Internet to find out more about the Data Protection Act 1998 and how it affects the beauty industry.

 Salon life

It was a very busy Saturday morning in the salon. The reception was buzzing with clients waiting for treatments and buying products. Li-ying noticed a woman hovering outside the door looking very unsure of herself. She wondered whether the woman wanted to see a brochure or book a treatment, or whether she was just waiting for someone. Li-ying wasn't sure what she should say to her.

Then Lisa, the salon junior, called to the woman over the heads of the other clients, saying 'Come in, we don't bite!' The woman came in rather sheepishly. Li-ying asked, 'How can we help?' The woman explained in a whispered voice that she was interested in waxing. 'What part of the body?' called out Lisa from the other end of the desk. The woman winced. She didn't want to say in front of all the other people, so took a brochure and hurried out saying that she would telephone later.

Could this matter have been dealt with better? If so, how?

Was the communication between the potential client and the staff good? Why?

Do you think that the woman will return to the salon? Give a reason for your answer.

? **Memory jogger**

1 What is confidential information?

2 Why must you store record cards or other confidential information in line with the Data Protection Act?

3 List three qualities and skills that are needed when dealing with complaints.

Help to make appointments for salon services [1]

One of your key tasks when assisting on reception will be to help make appointments. Booking appointments is not an easy thing to do. Mistakes can happen very easily, and very small mistakes in the appointment columns can cause huge problems for the salon staff, such as double bookings, lack of time to finish a treatment and clients left waiting. This can then result in a stressful environment where there are unhappy clients, overworked therapists and embarrassed staff.

Date: Tuesday 13th October 2009

	Lucy	Hellena	Anetta	Siobhan	
AM 9.00	Mrs Khan	Mrs Hughes			9.00 AM
9.15	full	full			9.15
9.30	Body wax	B/Massage			9.30
9.45	01234 45678	223335			9.45
10.00					10.00
10.15					10.15
10.30		Mrs Inder			10.30
10.45	Miss Jones	Pedicure			10.45
11.00	Aroma	+ ½ leg wax	Miss Westerby		11.00
11.15	Back massage	01235 771540	French		11.15
11.30	357928		Manicure		11.30
11.45			+ facial		11.45
12.00			01329 815242		12.00
12.15		Mrs Green		Mr. Vallete	12.15
12.30	LUNCH	Eye tint		Back massage	12.30
12.45		444321		+ pedicure	12.45
				02271 881570	
PM 1.00	Mr. Walsh				1.00 PM
1.15	Manicure		Miss Rudman		1.15
1.30	+back wax	LUNCH	Miss Allen	Miss Binder	1.30
1.45	02392 815815		x2 eyebows	waxing	1.45
2.00	Mrs Suling		335215	e/b + lip & chin	2.00
2.15	Eyebrow tidy	Miss Murphy	LUNCH	07807 577211	2.15
2.30	413927	Arm wax			2.30
2.45		+ u/arm wax			2.45
3.00		223792	Miss Nair	Mrs Pattel	3.00
3.15			Bridal	Sugaring	3.15
3.30		Miss Woolford	Top to toe	to x2 leg	3.30
3.45		Basic facial +	447 812	221 335	3.45
4.00	Mrs Wang	eye lash tint			4.00
4.15	Non-surg.	445 877			4.15
4.30	facial lift				4.30
4.45	08789 815 111				4.45
5.00		Mrs Townsend			5.00
5.15		M/up			5.15
5.30		lesson			5.30
5.45		315579 ext. 222			5.45
6.00					6.00
6.15					6.15
6.30					6.30
6.45					6.45
7.00					7.00

(Siobhan column note: lunchtime cover only)

A page from an appointment book

Booking basics

Salon appointments are recorded on loose sheets of paper, in an appointment book, or on an electronic record system on a computer. Paper appointment sheets contain several columns. At the top of each column, the name of the therapist is entered. The receptionist and other staff can then see clearly at a glance:

- which therapist is treating which client at which time
- which therapist has room for more appointments
- who is taking breaks and when.

The appointment pages are created or written up weeks in advance because appointments can be made months ahead, for example if a client is having a course of treatments. Another reason may be that a client wishes to book for a special occasion such as a pre-wedding pamper, and will therefore need to book a certain date and time months in advance. Writing up the weeks ahead also helps staff to plan their holidays and work timetables can then be organised around them.

Making a booking

A client may make a booking over the telephone, in person at the salon, by text or online. Electronic methods of booking are becoming much more popular.

The first thing you need to do is to take the client's details. You will need to find out the following.

- The client's surname and first initial. It is not advisable to write first names because other members of staff may not know the client by their first name, nor is it a good idea to just put a surname because there may be other clients with that name. If you write the client's first initial and surname, it is easy for a therapist to look up that person's details on a record card should they need to contact the client about the booking. Another reason for using the client's surname is that some clients do not like being called by their first name.
- The client's telephone number. Make sure that you write the dialing code if the telephone number is not a local one. You should also take down the client's work number if this is where the client can be contacted during working hours.
- The client's treatment. This is usually written in using an abbreviation.

Imagine if a first name only was entered into the appointment book, and the incorrect telephone number was written down. How could you try to contact the client to cancel her appointment if, for example, the therapist was ill?

If your salon uses an appointment book, follow this advice when writing in the columns.

- Appointments must be written in pencil only so that mistakes or changes can be rubbed out. Don't press too hard with the pencil as it makes it hard to rub out.
- Your writing should be neat, clear and small. This is to allow room for all the client and treatment details to be written in a small space.
- It is better to print words, rather than write in a joined up style, especially if your handwriting is not very good.

Top tip

If you are ever uncertain while helping on reception, ask for help. This is not a sign of failure; it shows that you are acting sensibly, and will help you to avoid making a double booking or an incorrect booking which then leads to an incorrect treatment.

> **Get up and go!**
>
> Design a client questionnaire to gain feedback from clients on how they think you performed while on reception duty. Make the questionnaire quite simple and short as clients may not have much time to complete it.

Identifying the client's requirements

When a client contacts you to make an appointment, let her tell you exactly what she would like before interrupting her. If the client only has an idea, then help her to decide. Then repeat the information to check that you have correctly understood her wishes. If you have the **authority** to book the treatment, then you can do so.

Help to make appointments for salon services (2)

Making a new booking

Here are the steps to booking an appointment in person or by telephone under the guidance of a senior staff member:

1 Ask what treatment the client would like to book and when.

2 Ask if the client would like to see a particular therapist.

3 Look at the appointment book and offer some available dates and times.

4 When the day, date and time have been agreed, write the client's name, telephone number and treatment in pencil only.

5 Read back the day, date, time and therapist to the client to make sure that no mistakes have been made. This part is very important.

6 Write down the appointment details on an appointment card to give to the client.

7 Get the senior member of staff to check the entry before the client leaves.

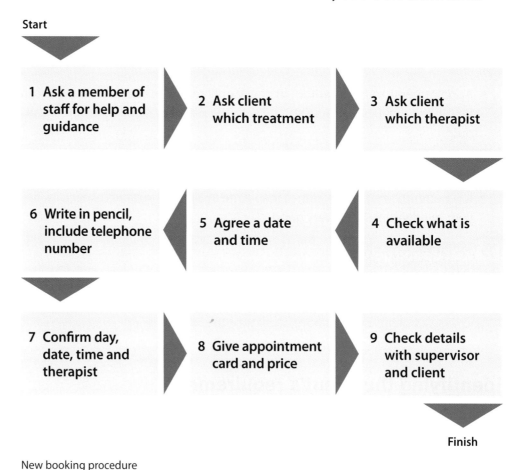

New booking procedure

When making an appointment, make sure that you write in the column as you confirm the day, date and time to a client. Never write this information in the column after putting down the telephone or after the client has left the salon – this is asking for trouble. Another client could come in, the phone could ring again, a senior therapist could ask you to do some jobs for her, by which time you will have forgotten all about the appointment that you should have written down.

What to do when problems arise:

- If the time that the client wants is not free, then offer the nearest time to it.

- If the client wants to see a certain therapist, but that therapist is already booked, then offer the client the next and nearest time available for that therapist. If that time is not convenient, then offer the client a different therapist.

- If an appointment needs to be changed, rub it out and rewrite it in the book and on the client's appointment card.

Booking out time for treatments

Another factor to think about is how long to book out for each treatment. Your manager will need to tell you how this is done for your salon, and show you how to do it. However, on nearly every appointment sheet, one line in a column stands for a 15-minute time slot. For example, if a facial takes one hour to complete, then four lines will need to be crossed through in a column.

When booking out some appointments, time should be allowed for client preparation, consultation, homecare and aftercare advice. You should therefore book out treatment time and add 15 minutes (one line) if needed. Examples are given in the table on page 95.

As a beauty therapist becomes more experienced at giving treatments, she will probably work more quickly and will not need all the time put aside for a treatment. She would therefore have enough time for preparation, consultation and advice, without the need for the receptionist to book out extra time for this. Extra time for preparation, consultation and advice is needed mainly for larger, more relaxing treatments such as facials, body massages and complementary therapies.

Help to make appointments for salon services (3)

Commercially acceptable treatment times

There are set times for treatments known as commercially acceptable treatment times. This is how long a treatment should take in order to make a salon money.

It is important to bear in mind these times when you are taking bookings. Some therapists work slightly slower or quicker than others, but still manage to complete their treatments within an acceptable time. Each therapist should let the receptionist know exactly how long she needs for each treatment.

More information on commercially acceptable treatment times can be found under Treatment times and prices on pages 320–321.

Treatment codes

As there is not much space for writing appointment details in the columns, abbreviated codes are used to show which treatment has been booked. These codes vary from salon to salon, but are usually quite similar. Treatment codes are shown in the last column of the table on page 95.

When not to book an appointment

It is rewarding to have responsibility, but remember that there is a limit to your **authority**. It is important that you do not carry out activities without the permission and guidance of a senior staff member. Appointment systems can be tricky to master and easy to mess up, so ask for help where necessary. Always check appointments with a senior staff member until you have been given permission to carry out bookings on your own.

However, there will be certain treatments or clients that you will never be allowed to book. Examples of these are given in the table below. Always pass these cases on to a senior member of staff.

When not to book a client	Reason why
A course of treatments	This needs careful thought and planning by the therapist carrying out the course of treatments, so the booking is best done by the therapist.
An electrical treatment such as electrolysis	More thorough consultation and advice are needed before a client is allowed to have electrical treatments. Sometimes a doctor's permission is needed.
A person under the age of 16 without a parent present	This is for insurance reasons and to check that the client has parental permission.
If a client cannot give you a contact telephone number	You would be unable to contact the client if there was a problem with the booking and you needed to change or cancel it, for example due to staff illness.
If a client comes in who has been disruptive and rude on a previous visit	A disruptive client will upset both staff and other clients.

Top tip ✓

If a client wishes to make an appointment when a senior staff member is busy, you will not have the authority to do this. Explain that you need help as you are learning. If you feel confident enough to make the booking, explain that you must get it checked afterwards.

⟫ Get up and go!

Copy and complete the table below to show lines to cross through and treatment codes. Complete this information for pedicure through to ear piercing.

Treatment	Maximum time allowed in minutes without consultation time	Preparation/consultation time	Number of lines to cross through in appointment sheet/book	Treatment code
Eyebrow shape	15 minutes	0 – advise while treating	1	EBS
Eyelash tint	20 minutes	0 – advise while treating	2	ELT
Facial	45 minutes	1 – for undressing, aftercare advice and tidying of work area	4	FAC
Make-up	45 minutes	0 – advise while treating	3	M-UP
Manicure	30 minutes	0 – advise while treating	2	MAN
Pedicure	45 minutes	1 – to allow drying time and putting on of shoes, also tidying of work area		
Eyebrow wax	15 minutes	0 – advise while treating		
Underarm wax	15 minutes	0 – advise while treating		
Half leg wax	30 minutes	0 – advise while treating		
Bikini wax	15 minutes	0 – advise while treating		
Arm wax	30 minutes	0 – advise while treating		
Full leg wax	50 minutes	0 – advise while treating		
Half leg, bikini and underarm wax	60 minutes	0 – advise while treating		
Full leg, bikini and underarm wax	75 minutes	0 – advise while treating		
Eyebrow shape and eyelash tint	35 minutes	0 – advise while treating		
Eyebrow tint	10 minutes	0 – advise while treating		
Eyelash tint, eyebrow tint and eyebrow shape	30 minutes	0 – advise while treating		
Ear piercing	15 minutes	0 – advise while treating		

? Memory jogger

1 Give two reasons why a client may not be treated.

2 How long would you book out for a half leg wax, bikini wax and eyebrow wax?

3 Why should you book the appointment while the client is still on the telephone or with you?

Getting ready for assessment

Evidence requirements

You will be observed by your assessor on at least three occasions, two of which will cover making appointments.

What you must cover during your practical assessments

Ranges

In your candidate handbook you will have a list of ranges that you must cover during your assessment. These ranges cover:

1 enquiries

2 methods of making appointments

3 appointment details.

From the range you must show that:

- you have demonstrated that you have dealt with face-to-face enquiries and telephone enquiries
- you have made appointments with a client face-to-face and by telephone
- your appointment details have covered clients, name and contact details, the service, the date, the time and the member of staff that will be carrying out the treatment or nail service.

It is good practice to cover as many ranges as possible during each assessment. This will prevent you having to take too many additional assessments because there are many ranges that you have not managed to cover.

Performance criteria

What you must demonstrate during a practical observation by your tutor:

- maintaining the reception area by keeping it clean and tidy
- keeping product displays neat, clean and tidy
- reporting low levels of stationery and retail to your supervisor
- offering clients hospitality
- attending to clients and enquiries
- recording messages and appointments accurately and **confidentially**
- showing good communication skills
- making and confirming appointments accurately.

Throughout your observations you will also need to make sure that you pay attention to health, safety and hygiene throughout, as well as presenting yourself well, so read through Unit G20 Make sure your own actions reduce risks to health and safety before any practical assessment just to refresh your memory.

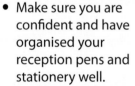

Top tips ✓

- Make sure you are confident and have organised your reception pens and stationery well.
- Prepare a checklist so that it is easy to check that you have everything to hand.
- Concentrate, don't let friends distract you.
- Be immaculately dressed with a ready smile on your face.

What you must know

In order to pass this unit, you will need to gather evidence during the teaching and learning of this unit before your assessor observes your practical performance. You will gather this during class work and further study and will probably file it in a portfolio of evidence. This evidence will also be signed off in your candidate handbook which you will be given by your assessor. This will be an official record to show that you have covered what you need to.

 Salon life

Sunita rushed into the salon, ten minutes late. Her bus had failed to arrive on time again.

It was Sunita's turn on reception today, and she hated it. She walked past two clients who were already waiting and dumped her handbag on the desk. Then she took out her make-up bag. She wanted to put her make-up on before her boss saw her. She was glad that no one caught her doing this. She eyed one of the women in the waiting area who was huffing and tutting. Sunita became annoyed. She always seemed to get lumbered with the awkward clients.

Janie, the head therapist, came into reception. She went straight to Sunita and told her off for not letting her know that her client had arrived. Sunita rolled her eyes – it was going to be one of those days. The phone rang. Sunita lifted the receiver but replaced it straight away, as she was not yet organised. She still needed to change into her uniform, put her bag in her locker and make a coffee to wake herself up.

Sunita went through to the staff room, where she chatted and giggled for a few minutes about the party she went to last night. Then she sorted herself out.

Sunita's day soon went from bad to worse. The salon manager called her into her office and gave her an oral warning about her conduct and attitude. She said that she was responsible for therapists starting treatments late, make-up on the appointment sheets and a theft in reception. To Sunita, this was terribly unfair. She was always the person who was blamed when anything went wrong. She decided that she would start looking for another job.

List the things that Sunita did wrong.

Comment on her attitude. Was it acceptable?

How could Sunita improve her morning routine and make herself a more popular staff member?

All about hair

What is hair?

Hair is made up of a protein called keratin. Your skin and nails are made from the same protein. A strand of hair is called a hair shaft, and it is made up of three layers: the cuticle, cortex and medulla.

Hair structure

The hair shaft is covered in overlapping cuticles, which can be thought of as being like fish scales or the tiles on a roof. When the hair is in good condition, the cuticles lie flat and when the hair is in bad condition the cuticles may be lifted or even torn away, exposing the cortex layer of the hair shaft.

Hair in good condition

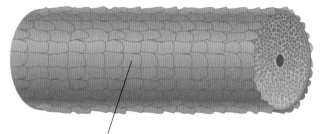

Cuticle scales lying close together

Hair in bad condition

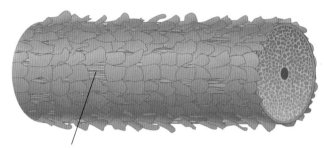

Cuticle scales open and misshapen. Some scales may have been completely destroyed, exposing the cortex

The effect of humidity on the hair is dependent on how well conditioned the hair shaft is and how flat, smooth and even the cuticle scales are. Hair is 'hygroscopic', which means that it absorbs moisture from the atmosphere. Hair that is porous will absorb moisture from the atmosphere more readily than hair that is non-porous. You should take great care when working on porous hair so as not to over-dry it. Directing airflow down the length of the hair shafts can help protect the cuticles.

 Get up and go!

Look at some different types of blow-drying products and consider their purposes. Think about products which can be used before and after the blow-dry. Create a chart of styling products and list the most suitable types of hair to use them on and what effects they will have. Show this information to your stylist or assessor and discuss the benefits of each product.

Cuticle

The outer layer is known as the cuticle layer of the hair shaft. The cuticle has overlapping scales wrapped around the centre of the hair known as the cortex. The hair when in good condition reflects the light and is smooth and shiny. The cuticle scales will also be tightly compacted giving a non-porous outer layer.

Cortex

The cortex layer of the hair shaft is made up of bundles of fibrils. Imagine a bundle of dried spaghetti or a bundle of pencils in your hand and this will reasonably reflect the structure of the cortex layer of the hair shaft. In the cortex we can see chemical changes altering the basic structure of the hair shaft. For example, when we perm the client's hair or apply a permanent colour we alter the basic structure of the hair. All chemical changes take place in the cortex. This includes bleaching, relaxing, permanent colouring and perming.

Medulla

The central layer of the hair is known as the medulla. It has no part to play in hairdressing treatments; it is simply made up of air spaces along the length of the hair shaft. The medulla may be present in some hairs but not in others, and may not be present for the full length of the hair.

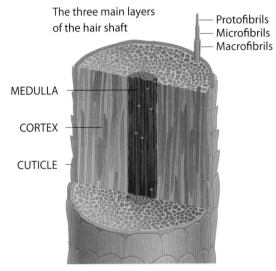

The three main layers of the hair shaft

— Protofibrils
— Microfibrils
— Macrofibrils

MEDULLA

CORTEX

CUTICLE

The hair shaft

Why do we have hair?

Protection

Hair has a protective function. If an object were to fall on your head the hair on your scalp would offer some, although limited, protection. The hair inside your nose acts as a filter when breathing, helping prevent dust and debris from entering your nasal passages, and your eyelashes offer some protection against dust entering your eyes.

Warmth

Hair acts as an insulator by helping keep the surface of the skin warm. You may notice when you are cold that hairs will stand up. This is the body's attempt to keep warm, by trapping a layer of warm air between the surface of the skin and the hair, which is standing up.

Looking good

How does your hair make you feel? Mostly when our hair looks good, we feel good! Hair offers a different dimension to how we feel about ourselves and how we can express ourselves. A freshly shampooed and well conditioned head of hair will give us an added confidence when compared with a head of hair which is greasy and in need of some tender loving care. Growth patterns of the hair may affect our choices of style, and you will need to consider the root direction of a client's hair when helping them select a style.

Different face shapes

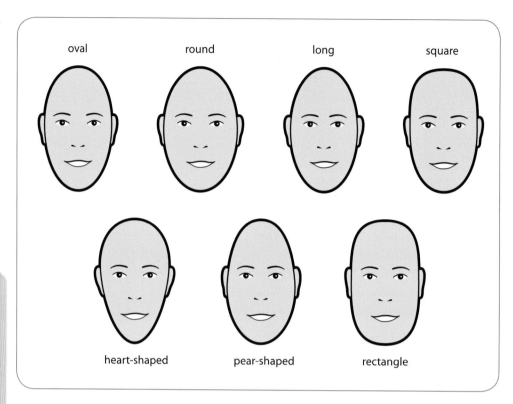

oval   round   long   square

heart-shaped   pear-shaped   rectangle

» Get up and go!

You are what you eat! As you have learned, hair is made up of a protein called keratin, and the basic building blocks of proteins are amino acids. We get these amino acids from the foods we eat, so you really can affect the condition of your hair with the types of food you eat. Think about the food you eat and the effect it might have on your hair. Hair loss and scalp problems can be caused by a poor diet and if our diet is poor, the likelihood is our hair will suffer.

Keep a food diary for one week, keeping a note of the food you eat and its nutritional value. Do you think you are getting enough protein, carbohydrates, vitamins and minerals to feed your body and your hair?

Your hair acts as a frame around your face, rather like a frame around a painting. And your hair can be styled to complement your face shape and to disguise less attractive features. Think about a client who may have a very wide forehead; would you give them a fringe?

Hair condition and hair types

Hair and scalp conditions can be divided into dry, normal, greasy and dandruff-affected.

Hair in good condition is soft to touch and hair in bad condition feels rough, dry and brittle. Hair can also be one of the following different types:

- Caucasian/European
- Asian/Oriental
- African type.

You will notice the hair is either straight or has an amount of natural wave or curl present.

- The Caucasian/European hair shaft can be straight, wavy or curly and its cross-section is oval shaped.
- The Asian/Oriental hair shaft can be straight and/or coarse and its cross-section is round.
- The African type hair shaft can be tightly or loosely curled and its cross-section is kidney shaped.

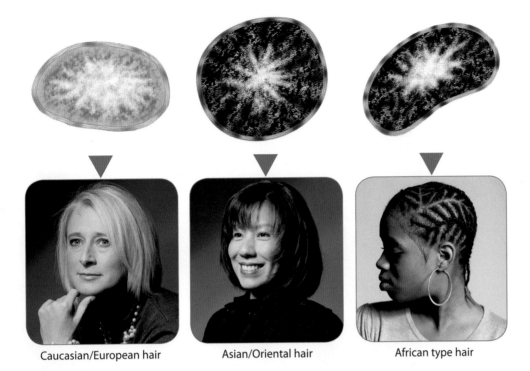

Caucasian/European hair   Asian/Oriental hair   African type hair

The texture of hair will vary from client to client and may also vary within the same head of hair. Texture can be fine, medium or coarse and is determined by touch.

Get ahead

Research the hair growth cycle as part of your preparation towards Level 2. Consider the follicle and how it widens at the bottom to encompass the papilla. Find out about the epidermal cells and how these are constantly growing and being pushed up towards the surface of the skin. Write a small project using the following headings and ask your assessor to look at it.

- Alpha and beta keratin
- How the cells change shape as they move along the hair follicle
- The cuticle, cortex and medulla
- Colour producing cells (melanocytes)
- The three stages of the hair growth cycle: anagen, catagen and telogen

Include photos and sketches to help the reader understand what you are explaining.

? Memory jogger

1 What protein is hair made of?

2 Name the three layers of the hair shaft.

3 What happens to the cuticles when hair is in either good or bad condition?

4 Where in the hair does chemical change take place during certain hairdressing services?

5 Why do we have hair?

6 Name the three different hair types and describe how they differ.

UNIT GH1

Shampoo and condition hair

The word 'shampoo' is a Hindustani word meaning 'to press or rub'. Shampooing and conditioning hair is one of the most important treatments in hairdressing. It prepares the hair for any treatments or services and can be the start of a pleasurable hairdressing experience for the client – or a complete disaster if carried out incorrectly!

This unit is about the skill of shampooing and conditioning the hair and scalp. You will learn about different massage techniques and some of the products available for different hair types. This unit applies to both ladies' and gents' hairdressing salons.

In this unit you will learn how to:

- Maintain effective and safe methods of working when shampooing and conditioning hair
- Shampoo hair
- Apply and remove conditioners.

Here are some key terms you may meet in this unit:

Minimise – reduce the effect of something

Friction – fast rubbing technique with a light plucking action

Products – shampoos, conditioners, styling sprays, creams and gels, etc.

Temperature – how hot or cold something is

Massage – manipulating the skin either manually or mechanically

Relevant person – assessor, stylist or line manager

Effleurage – slow, stroking, superficial movement, using the length of the hand

Rotary – penetrating, circular movement using the fingertips

Petrissage – slow, deep, penetrating circular movement using the fingertips

Surface conditioner – conditioner which lies on the outer layer of the hair shaft

Steamer – equipment providing moist heat, used during conditioning

Penetrating conditioner – conditioner which penetrates into the cortex layer of the hair shaft

Dermatitis – inflammation of the skin caused by an irritant

Maintain effective and safe methods of working when shampooing and conditioning hair [1]

Most people can shampoo their own hair at home and are likely to have done so many times. As a practising hairdresser, you will need to make sure your shampooing technique is of a high professional standard, and this will probably be a little different from how most people shampoo their own hair at home. The physical action of massaging a person's head can be invigorating, stimulating and relaxing. Be conscious of the person at your fingertips. Ask them how they like their hair and scalp to be shampooed.

Why shampoo hair?

We shampoo hair for three reasons.

- To remove excess natural oil, skin cells, dust and dirt.
- To remove the build-up of hair-care **products**.
- To prepare the hair for further treatments.

The success of the shampoo is important to the success of the following treatment, for example, the client's cut, perm or colour.

> **》 Get up and go!**
>
> Look at the various shampoos and conditioners in your salon. Now complete the table below matching the products in your salon with the hair types. This information will be useful when offering clients professional advice about their hair and scalp condition.
>
> | Hair/scalp type | Shampoo | Conditioner |
> |---|---|---|
> | Coloured | Colour preserver | Colour preserver |
> | Fine | | |
> | Permed | | |
> | Normal | | |
> | Dry/damaged | | |
> | Dandruff-affected | | |
> | Oily | | |

Preparation

Your salon's requirements for client preparation should include a thorough hair and scalp analysis by an experienced stylist who will confirm whether it is safe for you to carry out the treatment.

Protecting the client

The client's clothing must be protected at all times. Always use a clean gown and towel. If the client is not gowned properly, their clothing may get wet, or even damaged if they are having a chemical treatment.

Positioning the client and checking your posture

Position the client correctly at either the back-wash or front-wash basin and check your client is comfortable. The client's position will affect how you stand at the basin and how tired you will feel at the end of the shampoo. Poor posture may have a long-term effect on your wellbeing, so make sure your position and posture during the shampoo **minimises** the risk of tiredness and injury to yourself.

> ### » Get up and go!
>
> Practise preparing a colleague for a shampoo with a gown, towel and a waterproof cape. Consider how claustrophobic it may make you feel if everything is too tight. Remember to allow some room for your client to breathe – it can get warm under those protective layers. Always ask the client if they are comfortable.
>
> Now find out how to prepare a client for the following services and practise on your colleague: perming; relaxing; colouring; cutting; setting.

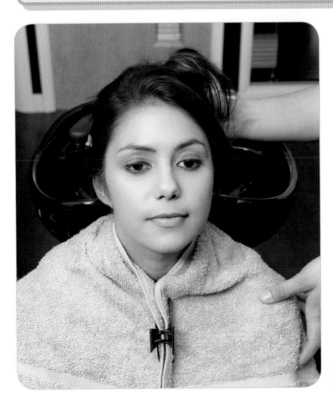

Position the client comfortably at a back-wash basin

? Memory jogger

1 Why do we shampoo hair?
2 What are the effects of having poor posture whilst shampooing your clients?
3 What products would you recommend for a client who has oily hair?
4 Why should you always gown a client correctly before carrying out any treatment?
5 What should be carried out before any hairdressing treatment begins?
6 What products would you recommend for a client with dry hair?

Maintain effective and safe methods of working when shampooing and conditioning hair (2)

Working methods

Using resources efficiently

Resources such as hairdressing **products** are expensive and it is important to use them cost-effectively. Some shampoos have pump dispensers and these may help to reduce unnecessary waste by dispensing just the right amount of product. By minimising waste you save money, therefore making the salon a more profitable business.

Reducing the risk of cross-infection

Any tools or equipment that come into contact with clients' hair and skin must be completely clean. This will help to maintain a safe and hygienic working environment. As well as keeping the salon clean, you must always remember your personal cleanliness. Make sure your own standards of health and hygiene help to reduce the risk of cross-infection. For example, do not come into the salon if you have a cold or contagious disease, or an infestation such as head lice. Stay at home and minimise the risk of cross-infection; when the condition has cleared, it is then safe to return to work. By ensuring your personal standards of health and hygiene you **minimise** the risk of cross-infection, infestation and offence to your clients and colleagues.

Reducing the risk of injury

Your hands are essential to carrying out everyday tasks both in the workplace and at home. As your hands will often be in water, always dry them thoroughly and use a barrier cream and protective gloves. This will help to reduce the risk of contact **dermatitis**, a skin condition which often affects hairdressers. It is caused by constant contact with products, such as shampoos and chemicals. Should the condition worsen, you should seek medical advice.

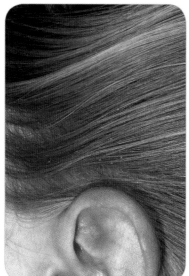

Head lice hatch from eggs called nits. They can be found on the hair shaft close to the scalp

> **» Get up and go!**
>
> Next time you are in the salon, discreetly observe how many staff are wearing jewellery on their hands. It is best to leave your rings at home. This will make it easier for you to clean your hands properly and help prevent dermatitis. Ask your colleagues if they have ever suffered from dry, itchy hands or dermatitis.

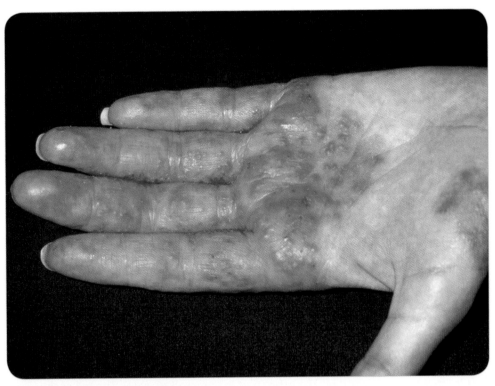

Protect your hands against dermatitis

It is essential to store, use, handle and dispose of products in accordance with manufacturers' instructions, salon policy and local bylaws. When dealing with resources in the salon, you will be expected to have a good working knowledge of the Control of Substances Hazardous to Health (COSHH) Regulations, therefore minimising the risk of harm or injury to yourself and others.

Re-filling and re-ordering products

Shampoos, conditioners and chemical products are in constant use in the salon.

Keep a look out for opportunities to replenish low levels of resources, when required, to minimise disruption to your own work and to clients. Should you notice that the stock level of any product is running low and needs re-ordering, report it to the **relevant person**.

> **» Get up and go!**
>
> With a colleague, think of reasons why shampoo and conditioner dispensers need to be regularly filled up and why stock levels of products need to be checked regularly. What might the effects be if the salon runs out of something? Who should stock shortages be reported to in your salon?

> **? Memory jogger**
>
> 1 What are the appropriate measures for disposing of chemicals in the salon?
> 2 Why should you re-fill products on a regular basis?
> 3 What does COSHH stand for?
> 4 Describe how dermatitis can be prevented.
> 5 How can you use resources cost-effectively?

Shampooing hair (1)

How long should a shampooing and conditioning treatment take?

Depending on the length and thickness of the client's hair, a basic shampoo and surface condition in industry should take 3–5 minutes. You might find it helpful to watch your colleagues and time them, making sure they make effective use of their working time. You must practise with:

- above shoulder-length hair, for assessment purposes this should take a maximum of 10 minutes
- below shoulder-length hair, for assessment purposes this should take a maximum of 15 minutes.

How shampoo works

Shampoo comes in many types, consistencies, colours and aromas. It mixes easily with water allowing grease, dirt and oil to be rinsed out of the hair. It works because it contains detergent molecules. Each detergent molecule consists of two parts – one part is attracted to dirt and oil, the other part is attracted to water. The tail of the detergent molecule digs into the dirt and oil on the surface of the hair and scalp. The head of the detergent molecule has a negative electric charge. As a result of **massage** movements, dirt and oil is repelled from the hair and rinsed away in the water.

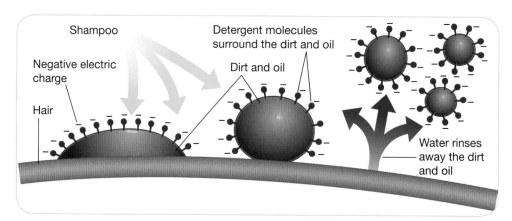

How detergent molecules in shampoo cleanse the hair

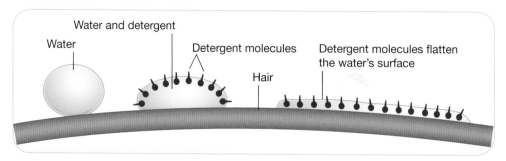

Shampoo flattens the surface tension of the water

Water also has a high surface tension, which has the effect of producing a 'skin' on the surface of the water. Shampoos flatten the surface tension of water making it easier to shampoo the client's hair.

How conditioner works

Hair is made of a protein called keratin. The same protein is found in skin and nails.

Hair in poor condition may have been damaged by overuse of heated styling equipment, incorrect brushing or too many chemical treatments. Conditioners strengthen and moisturise the hair.

There are many types of conditioner. They include the following:

- **Surface conditioner** coats the hair shaft and smoothes down the cuticle scales leaving the hair tangle-free.
- Anti-oxidant conditioner prevents any further oxidation to the hair shaft after chemical treatments.
- Specialist treatment conditioners strengthen the hair shaft internally by filling the air spaces caused by damage with liquid protein. This gives the hair added elasticity, sheen and manageability.
- Almond or olive oils are used mainly for dry scalps.

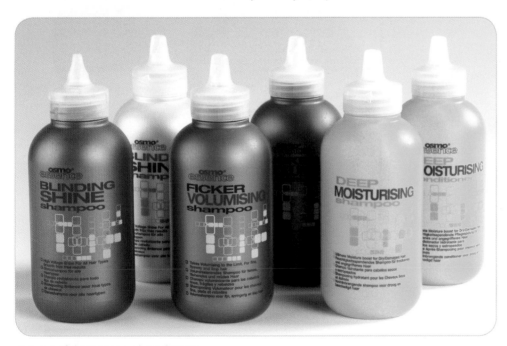

A range of shampoos and conditiners

? Memory jogger

1 How long should a shampoo and conditioning treatment take to complete?
2 Briefly explain how shampoo works.
3 What protein is hair made from?
4 What might cause hair to become damaged?
5 Why might you use an almond or olive oil to treat hair?

Shampooing hair (2)

Working with the stylist

There are many different levels of staff within a salon, including:

- staff who shampoo and carry out basic skills
- staff who practise technical skills like perming, relaxing, cutting and colouring
- senior staff who may manage the salon.

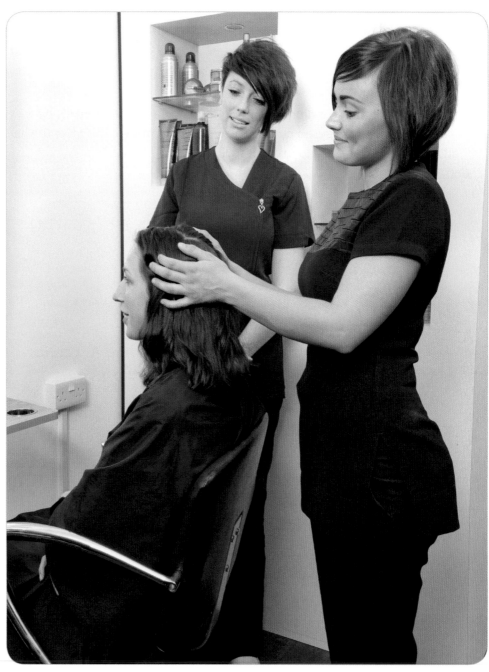

An experienced stylist instructs a junior member of staff

Part of your job role will involve learning to work with people and take instructions from senior colleagues. They may ask you to use a product in a particular way, or to change your massage movements to suit a different hair type and length. Following their advice and listening to the information they give will help you develop within your job role.

Using products and tools

Acid and alkali products

Acid and alkali products are regularly used in the salon. **Acid products** include perms, colours, shampoos, conditioners, bleach and peroxide. Acid-based conditioners are considered to be kinder to the hair because they close down the cuticle scales and return the pH of hair to pH 4.5–5.5. They also help maintain moisture within the hair shaft and give a smooth, shiny, tangle-free finish to the hair.

Alkali products include bleach, colours, perms, relaxers and some shampoos. These products lift the cuticle scales and give a roughened feel and appearance to the outer layer of the hair shaft. The pH of most hair when chemically treated is often more than pH 7, which is why the hair must be returned to its natural acid state of pH 4.5–5.5.

Steamers

A **steamer** produces a constant amount of steam contained within a hood. The hood is similar to that of a hood hairdryer. It works rather like a kettle. You will use a steamer to help:

- the penetration of conditioner
- replace lost moisture
- strengthen the internal and external layer of the hair shaft.

You should only use a steamer if you have been trained in how to do so and, as with all salon products, you should always follow the stylist's instructions in accordance with the manufacturer's instructions. The Electricity at Work Regulations cover the safe use of electrical equipment in the salon, including steamers (see Unit G20 for more information on these regulations).

First, fill the reservoir with distilled (not tap) water. This is to make sure no impurities coat the element and block the tiny water valves. With dry hands, plug in and switch on the steamer. While you **massage** the client's hair and scalp, the water will heat up and release steam into the hood. Place the client under the hood for 5–10 minutes. Remember to offer the client a drink or a magazine to read. When the time is up, take the client out from under the steamer. Switch off and unplug the steamer. Clean the steamer as soon as you have finished with it, leaving it ready for the next client.

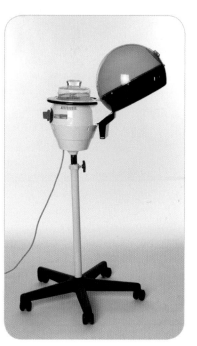

A steamer

Shampooing hair (3)

Water temperature and flow

The **temperature** of the water plays an important part in cleansing the hair and scalp. The flow of water is important too. Both the temperature and flow you use will depend on the amount of hair the client has and the sensitivity of their scalp. Very hot water will burn the client's scalp, but if the water is not hot enough, the hair will not be fully cleansed. There are times when you may need to use tepid (warm) water. For example, if the client's hair and scalp are oily, tepid water will help the sebaceous glands to produce less sebum (oil) when carrying out a light massage during the shampoo.

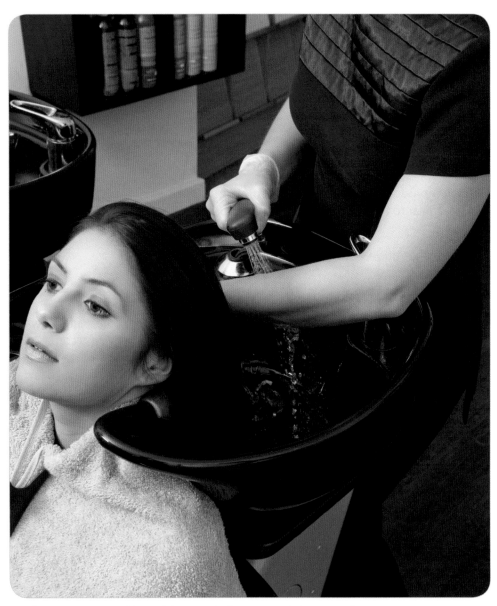

Test the temperature and flow of the water before you apply it to your client

Before and during each shampoo, it is essential to test the temperature of the water, either on the back of your hand or on the inside of your wrist. Remember to check the temperature of the water is comfortable for your client regularly. Adapt the water temperature, flow and direction to suit the needs of your client's hair and the next part of the service. Always turn the tap off between shampoos. Hot water is too expensive to simply let run down the plughole!

Choosing shampoo

You will need to choose the most appropriate shampoo for the client's hair and scalp condition. Some treatments that follow a shampoo may not need a conditioner. For example, when perming a client's hair, conditioner will coat the cuticle and act as a barrier, giving an unsatisfactory result. Make sure you know which shampoo to use (go back to the table you completed on page 104 to remind yourself).

Be careful not to spill shampoo, but if you do, you will need to clear up any spillages straight away for the safety of your client, colleagues and yourself.

>> **Get up and go!**

Take a look at the different hairstyles worn by colleagues at your salon. Some styles work better if the hair is not shampooed very often. Other styles need a regular shampoo. Create a simple list of hairstyles which require less frequent shampooing and hairstyles that require more frequent shampooing.

? **Memory jogger**

1 What is the natural pH of hair?

2 Why is a steamer used?

3 What type of water would you use in a steamer?

4 What massage movements are commonly used when conditioning?

5 Which massage movements are used mainly when shampooing?

6 When might you use tepid water to shampoo and condition a client's hair? Why?

Shampooing hair [4]

Massage techniques

During the shampoo and application of conditioner, you will need to use certain massage movements. The most popular movements used within the salon are:

- **effleurage**
- **rotary**
- **petrissage.**

The amount of shampoo you use for each client will be different depending on the length and thickness of their hair. A small amount of shampoo, no bigger than the size of a ten pence piece, is usually sufficient. Dispense the shampoo into the palm of your hand. Rub both palms together and then place the palms of your hands on the client's hair, smoothing the shampoo on to the scalp and down the hair length.

You can now use the massage movements. For a thorough shampoo and conditioning treatment, make sure your massage techniques achieve an even distribution of product over the hair and scalp. Take care not to pull your client's hair or scratch their scalp. This will cause irritation and discomfort to your client and may prevent the next part of the hair service from being carried out.

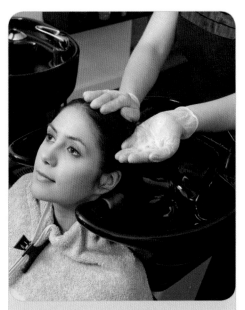

1   Effleurage movement

Effleurage is used to spread the shampoo throughout the hair at the start of the shampoo and each time you repeat the application of shampoo. Effleurage is a light, slow and superficial movement used as a linking movement to rotary massage.

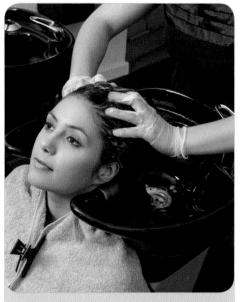

2   Rotary massage

Rotary massage is used during the shampoo. It is much deeper and faster than effleurage. Your hands should be claw-like when positioned on the client's scalp and should move in small, fast, circular movements with a firm pressure.

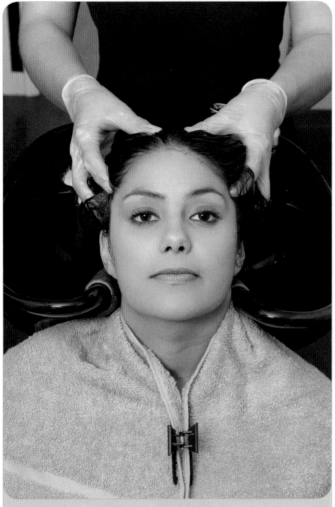

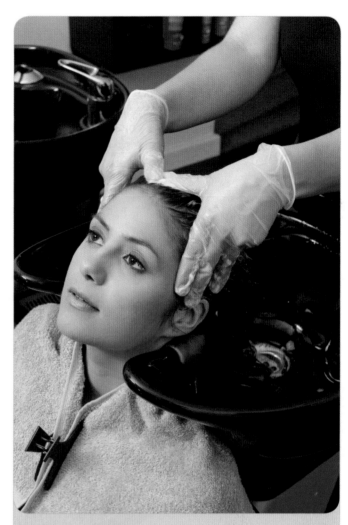

3   Petrissage movement

Petrissage is a slower version of the rotary movement and is used when carrying out a conditioning treatment. It should totally relax the client, assist penetration of the conditioner and promote blood circulation. Petrissage helps to make the hair smooth, shiny and manageable.

4   Friction massage

Friction is a massage movement that involves a fast rubbing technique and has a light, gentle plucking action. It is sometimes used when shampooing or when applying lotions such as astringents.

» Get up and go!

Find out from a colleague at your salon what an astringent is and what it is used for.

Applying and removing conditioners (1)

When you have completed the shampoo, you may have to apply conditioning products using the effleurage and petrissage massage movements. Always apply conditioners to the hair following the stylist's and manufacturer's instructions. A conditioning treatment will smooth down the cuticle scales, maintain moisture levels, protect and promote shine and improve the feel of the hair.

When removing conditioning products it is important to:

- avoid disturbing the direction of the cuticle
- comb through your client's hair without causing damage to the hair and scalp
- leave your client's hair free of excess water and product.

Should any problems occur, speak promptly to the **relevant person** in your salon.

After you have finished shampooing and conditioning, rinse the hair thoroughly. This is important to the success of the following treatment. Stylists do not want to ask their client to return to the basin to have excess product removed from the hair. Towel-dry the hair and wrap it in a towel, using a turban style. If you have used a steamer, rinse the client's hair with cooler water than you shampooed with. This will help to smooth down the cuticle scales of the hair ready for styling.

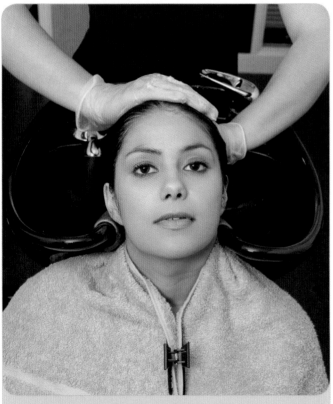

1   Using effleurage massage when applying conditioner

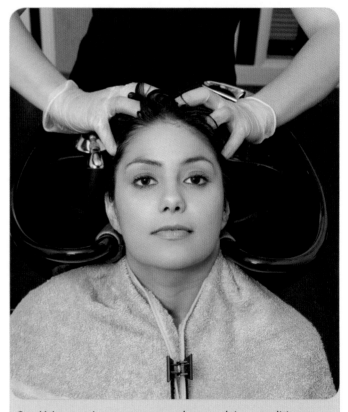

2   Using petrissage massage when applying conditioner

Applying and removing conditioners (2)

Completing the shampooing and conditioning treatment

The stylist will need you to leave the client's hair free of excess moisture and tangle-free. You will need to comb through from the points to the roots of the hair, without causing any damage to the hair and scalp in preparation for the next treatment.

The client will welcome any advice or guidance you can offer about how to maintain their newly conditioned hair at home. Always be knowledgeable about the products your salon sells. Discuss with your client, at the consultation stage and at the basin, the suitability of professional shampoo and conditioning products. This will help maintain the moisture level of your client's hair and offer protection in between salon visits, particularly if they are having a chemical treatment such as a colour or a perm.

If a client tells you they are shortly going on a beach holiday, advise them to pack hair-care products such as sunscreen, leave-in conditioner and moisturising shampoo. In addition, they can help protect their hair by covering it with a sun hat and removing all traces of chlorine and sea water as soon as possible after swimming.

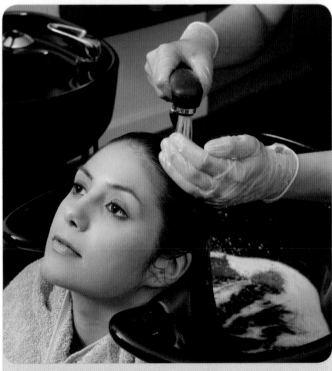

1 Make sure that you rinse the client's hair free of conditioner

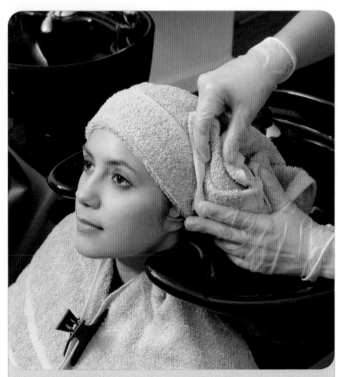

2 Wrap the client's hair in a towel using a turban style

≫ Get up and go!

With a colleague, create a list of the physical and chemical treatments an average head of hair may experience, considering how conditioning treatments may be able to help in each case.

? Memory jogger

1 What temperature of water would you choose to rinse off a conditioning treatment?

2 Why is the flow of water important when shampooing and conditioning?

3 Why is it important to comb the client's hair from points through to roots following a shampoo and conditioning treatment?

4 When would you choose not to apply a conditioner?

5 Why remove excess moisture from the client's hair following the shampoo and condition?

6 What advice might you give a client going on a beach holiday about looking after their hair?

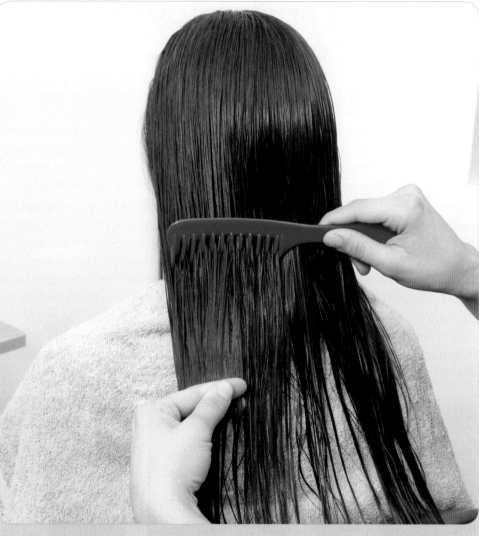

3 Comb through the client's hair, leaving it ready for the next service

⬆ Get ahead

Now you know how shampoos and conditioners can affect the hair, you might want to learn a little about how water affects hair. Did you know there are two different types of water: hard and soft? Each can affect hairdressing considerably. One can be more damaging than the other, particularly to the electrical equipment that steams or heats the water.

Find out which type of water area you work in and how this type of water can affect hairdressing. If you are in a hard water area, what measures can you take to prevent the build up of limescale? Write up your findings and present them to your colleagues. Can you make it into a mini-teaching session?

Step-by-step shampooing and conditioning

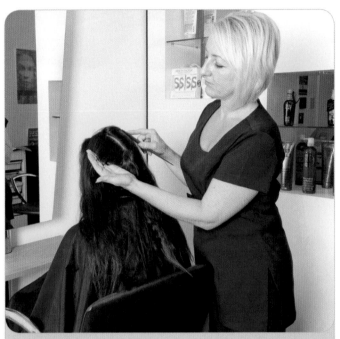

1. Gown up the client and analyse her hair and scalp before shampooing

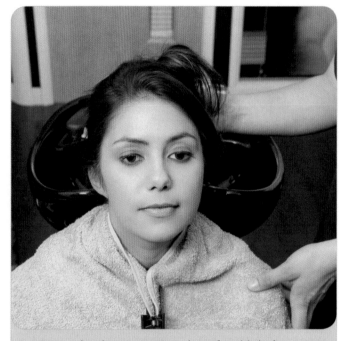

2. Ensure the client is positioned comfortably before shampooing

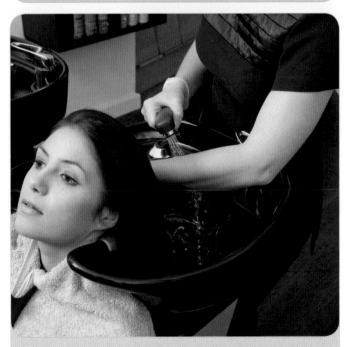

3. Test the temperature of the water before wetting the client's hair

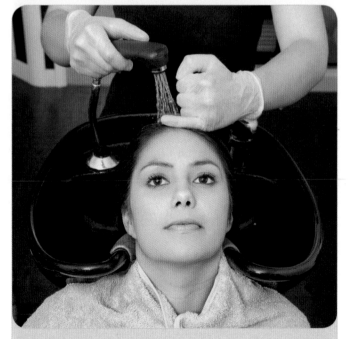

4. Apply the water to the client's hair, taking care not to wet her face

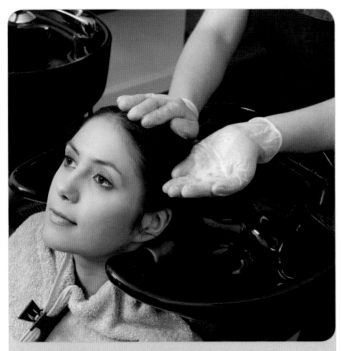

5 Using **effleurage massage**, apply the shampoo

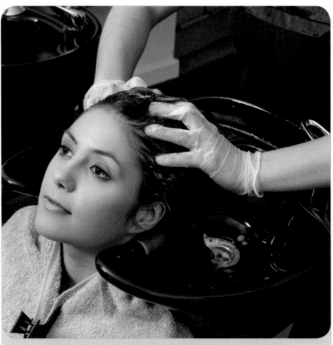

6 Use **rotary massage** over the whole head until the shampoo lathers and then rinse the hair free from shampoo

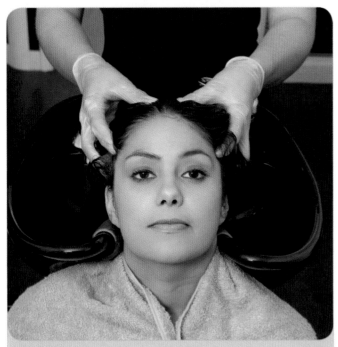

7 Apply the conditioner using both effleurage and **petrissage** movements. Rinse the conditioner from the hair and turn off the water. Wrap the client's hair in a towel

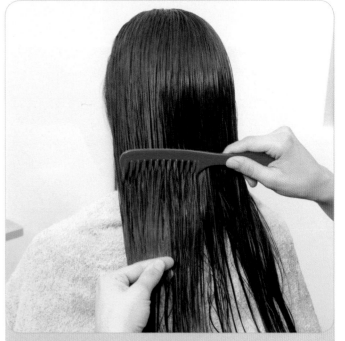

8 Squeeze the hair to remove excess water. Place a towel around the client's shoulders to prevent any drips and comb through the client's hair ready for further treatment

Getting ready for assessment

Evidence requirements

You will be observed by your assessor on at least three occasions, this must involve all massage techniques, all hair lengths, and all types of conditioning products. This unit also includes an external paper.

What you must cover during your practical assessments

Ranges

In this unit you must have covered the ranges below:

1 above and below shoulder length hair

2 effleurage, rotary and petrissage massage techniques

3 surface and treatment conditioning products.

Performance criteria

In order to perform this unit successfully you must:

- maintain effective and safe methods of working when shampooing and conditioning hair
- shampoo hair using appropriate products and massage techniques
- adapt water temperature and direction to suit the needs of the client
- leave the client's hair tangle free
- leave the client's hair free of product build up, shampoo and excess water
- apply conditioners to the hair by appropriate products and massage techniques
- remove conditioning products in a way that avoids disturbing the direction of the cuticle
- refer any problems to the relevant person promptly.

What you must know

In order to pass this unit, you will need to gather evidence to support a consistent performance with colleagues and clients. You should also collect evidence to show that you have taken part in self development activities over a period of time. This evidence will be signed off in your candidate handbook which you will be given by your assessor. This will be an official record to show that you have covered what you need to.

UNIT GH3

Prepare for hair services and maintain work areas

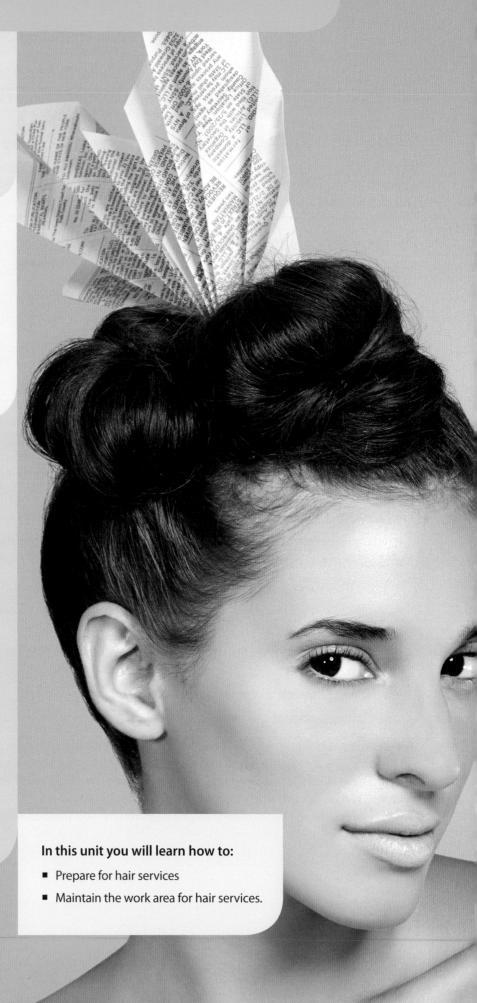

When working in the salon, one of your main duties will be preparing clients for services and setting up products, tools and equipment for stylists. Regularly checking what services and treatments are booked, knowing what is needed for each of them and being able to tidy away and clean up properly afterwards are essential skills.

You will need to demonstrate that you can meet the standards for preparing and maintaining hairdressing work areas. Following certain health, safety and hygiene procedures will become a normal part of your day-to-day duties. Everything you have learned so far about health and safety and COSHH needs to be brought together in this unit. Go back to Unit G20 to remind yourself of the health and safety aspects of working in a salon. Your assessor will observe your performance, which must include preparation for different hairdressing treatments, such as ladies' or gents' hairdressing services.

In this unit you will learn how to:

- Prepare for hair services
- Maintain the work area for hair services.

Here are some key terms you may meet in this unit:

Materials –
resources you will need to carry out a client's treatment

Dispose –
the correct removal of unwanted materials, products and other salon waste

Consultation –
a meeting with a client to talk about and decide with them what they want from a treatment

Stock –
products, materials and resources needed for clients' treatments

Records –
client details held either manually (on paper) or electronically (on computer)

Service –
what you have given your client by way of your help, time and expertise, e.g. cut, blow dry, colour, perm, etc.

Prepare for hair services (1)

Start as you mean to go on

Preparing for hair **services** isn't just about getting tools and equipment ready. Think about the type of people who may come through your salon door. Are they busy working people with little time on their hands? Are they parents with young children? Are they able-bodied or disabled? Notice your clients' body language as they enter the salon. Do they look rushed, frustrated, or perhaps calm?

You can begin to prepare for a client's hair service as soon as they enter the salon. If you notice a client has difficulty walking or moving around, or has a pushchair or shopping bags, find out if they need help coming into the salon. You may be able to hold the door for them, move things out of their way, or help them to a chair. Try to remember what help your client needed so you can be ready to offer it again next time they visit. Demonstrate a patient, positive attitude and make sure your body language is always professional.

≫ Get up and go!

Here are a few different services and treatments your salon may have booked on a regular basis:

Service/treatment	Products, tools and equipment needed
Setting	
Blow-drying	
Perming	
Colouring	
Cutting	
Straightening	
Hair-up	
Plaiting	
Hair extensions	
Shaving	
Beard trimming	

Copy out the table and for each service list in the right-hand column the products, tools and equipment that will be required. Don't forget things like cotton wool, disposable gloves and barrier cream, and whether or not you will need to set up a trolley.

Now practise setting up trays with a colleague. Check each other's trays and find out if you have both included everything you need.

Setting up materials, tools and equipment

Think about the most sensible way in which to set up **materials**, tools and equipment for the hair **services** offered by your salon. What clients do you have booked in today? You will need to check the appointment book, see what **stock** is required for each service and check you have the necessary items in the stock room. Discuss each client's requirements with your stylist.

Gowns and towels, and tools and equipment required for popular hairdressing treatments, must always be readily available. This will present a professional image and help save time for you and the stylist. The client will also be able to have their treatment completed in good time, making the visit a cost-effective one for the salon and an enjoyable one for the client.

As each of the services your salon offers has its own particular requirements in terms of resources, you need to be thorough in your preparation. It is particularly important to check all electrical equipment is in good working order, clean and fit for its purpose. Similarly, are products good to use? Check for any punctures or leaks in tubes and containers, and whether lids have been replaced properly. For example, the stylist will need the following if a perm is booked:

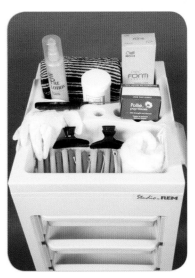
Perming trolley set up ready for stylist

- disposable gloves
- plastic apron
- combs
- section clips
- different-sized rods
- end papers
- cotton wool
- tension strips
- plastic cap
- barrier cream
- the appropriate perming lotion and neutraliser
- manufacturer's instructions.

? Memory jogger

1 What types of people may come through your salon door?

2 How do you know what to set up for each treatment your salon offers?

Prepare for hair services (2)

Preparing in good time

The tools, equipment and work area that stylists use need to be ready in time for the required treatment. Constantly think ahead and prepare the area as necessary for your stylist and, ultimately, your client. Be alert for signs that your team may need something, such as a comb or pair of clippers. Watch what each staff member uses – he or she may have a favourite comb or brush. Does this need to be sterilised before the next client?

Look at the appointment book on a regular basis so that you know what work is planned for the day. Bear in mind appointments might change during the day and you need to know the status of the appointment book at any one time. This means you need to liaise constantly with the receptionist to make sure changes are being passed on to you.

Now think about the type of work that has been booked in for the day. There may be several perms, some colours, a relaxer and a conditioning treatment. You will need to prepare for each treatment separately. Sometimes it is a good idea to check the appointments the day before, especially with chemical treatments. Check you have the necessary perms, relaxers and colours required for each of the clients.

Observe and anticipate

As you become more knowledgeable about hairdressing skills and get to know your colleagues, you will be able to observe what is happening in the salon and anticipate when your help is needed. Observation plays a major part in many hairdressing salons. Staff can 'speak' to each other using eye contact rather than words. Be alert to the signs that you may be needed and learn to identify your team's body language. This will help you anticipate the needs of other people, which in turn will benefit both clients and colleagues. Remember though to observe, not stare! Make sure that when you watch someone it is for a professional purpose.

At the end of a treatment

Timing in the salon is everything – sometimes things can happen too soon or not soon enough. Think about the products that may be needed at the end of a treatment. It could be serum, hairspray, wax, or a mixture of different products. Be on the look out for opportunities to assist your team as they are finishing off their clients.

Client records

Record cards are a professional record of what has been applied to your clients' hair. They are also a useful tool for recording positive comments and suggestions for any future treatment the client may request. The personal and professional information held on the record card is protected by the Data Protection Act. It is very important for record cards to be stored correctly in a lockable cabinet. Do you know what year the Data Protection Act came into force?

When obtaining **records** for your stylist's client, always remember to check the name, address and telephone number. Clients may share the same surname and even the same first name, and you don't want to give the stylist the wrong information.

 Salon life

Client record cards hold detailed information from past treatments. This information is crucial to the success of any hairdressing treatment. Imagine a situation where a stylist is off sick. Would another stylist know what was previously used on the client? Do you remember all of the products, mixes, timings and results from past clients?

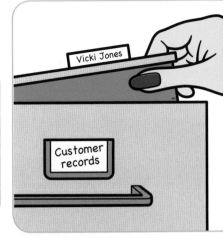

Clients' record cards must be stored properly in a locked cabinet

Records are important, to both your salon and your clients. They inform you of the products used previously, the timing and what the client's thoughts were regarding the result. Always have the client's record card ready in time for the **consultation** by the stylist. Clear away and file record cards as soon as they have been finished with. Your next client does not want the previous client's colour applied to his or her hair.

 Get up and go!

Think of a retail incentive scheme where all staff are encouraged to sell retail products and more chemical and non-chemical treatments. This could lead to greater income for the salon and perhaps a higher return for all staff in terms of an increased salary.

Look at the retail chart below and think of a way in which all staff could benefit, from the junior to the senior manager.

Staff name	Week 1	Week 2	Week 3	Week 4
Sylvia				Straighteners
Sue	Conditioning mousse	Moisturising shampoo	Scrunchie	
Jane		Brush	Serum	
Charmaine	Hair shine		Chemical treatment	

At the end of week 4, the salon could simply total the cost of sales and reward the member of staff who sold the most. Some hairdressing companies donate gifts as retail incentives. Discuss this system with a senior member of staff at your next staff meeting.

? Memory jogger

1 Why is timing important when setting out materials and products for your stylist?

2 What could you check against to find out what stock is needed for the day ahead?

3 Where should record cards be kept?

4 What does 'confidential' mean?

5 For whose benefit are record cards kept?

Prepare for hair services [3]

Cleaning the work area and sterilising tools and equipment

Remember to clear away all **materials**, tools and equipment when the stylist has finished with them. Wipe down the styling area with a suitable cleansing liquid at the most appropriate time and make sure the area is hair-free. Think about how you would feel if a stylist used a comb on your hair that had been used on clients all day without being cleaned and sterilised.

Salons are breeding grounds for bacteria. Make sure all equipment is clean for every client. Combs, brushes and all tools and equipment that have come into contact with the client's hair and scalp must be cleaned and sterilised ready for the next client. Sterilising destroys all living organisms. You may also use disinfectants in the salon to clean work areas. Disinfecting slows down the growth of bacteria.

Methods of sterilisation

Different tools and equipment need to be sterilised using different methods. For example, soft plastics cannot withstand the heat of an autoclave (which reaches 125°C) and will change shape or simply melt – a plastic roller will come out looking like a chewed piece of gum! Be careful to choose the right method for each piece of equipment. Take advice and guidance from the stylist or senior manager on how to sterilise correctly.

The three most commonly used methods of sterilising salon tools and equipment are:

- barbicide
- ultraviolet cabinet
- autoclave.

Barbicide is often used for sterilising combs and scissors and should be changed daily. An ultraviolet cabinet can sterilise small pieces of equipment made of plastic, such as brushes, combs and section clips. Autoclaves will sterilise objects made of rubber and metals, such as good quality combs and scissors.

Remember that all tools and equipment must be cleaned before sterilising. For example, use warm soapy water for combs, brushes, rollers etc. Wipe metal scissors with a suitable wipe and make sure scissors and clipper attachments are hair free.

≫ Get up and go!

Make a list of the different types of sterilisation methods available in your salon. Find out how each one works and what tools they are used to sterilise.

Salon life

What happens during a day in the life of a hairdresser? Think about your working day from start to finish and all the things you do. Many of them you probably do automatically and don't even think about. Maybe some of your colleagues aren't aware of all the things you do and how varied they are.

Make a list of all the tasks you do on an average day. Look at the list and think about how important each task is to the smooth running of the salon. Some of the things you do may be mundane, but if you didn't do them, life in the salon for your colleagues would soon become difficult.

Why not discuss your list at your next review or staff meeting? You may enlighten some people about what you do and ultimately surprise them!

? Memory jogger

1 What is the difference between disinfecting and sterilising?

2 Name three methods of sterilisation used in a salon.

3 What temperature does an autoclave reach?

Maintain the work area for hair services (1)

Disposing of hair and waste materials safely

The correct **disposal** of hair and waste materials is vital to the success of your salon. This isn't just to keep the salon looking clean and tidy – an Environmental Health Officer can, and often does, close down salons where staff have failed to deal with salon waste correctly.

Removing hair and waste from the salon means following health and safety procedures and using controlled and environmentally friendly methods. Here are some aspects of waste management you should be aware of.

- Loose hair should be cleared from basins to prevent blockages.
- Empty conditioner or shampoo bottles should be put in a plastics bin.
- Any left-over tint, bleach or perm lotion should be poured down the basin.
- Cut hair from the salon floor should be incinerated (burned) and disposed of by the local authority.
- Sharp items such as razor blades should be stored in a sharps box, which is then disposed of by a specialist company.
- Hairspray and mousse containers must be disposed of by a recognised company.

Removing waste quickly and correctly will give clients a professional image of the salon. It also reduces the risk of injury and cross-infection by keeping your work area clean and tidy during the service.

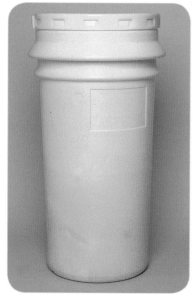

A sharps bin is the only way to dispose of items like razor blades

The Control of Substances Hazardous to Health (COSHH) Regulations (2002)

The COSHH Regulations greatly affect the way in which salons dispose of their waste by setting out basic measures employers and employees must take. In addition, each local authority has its own policy on how to deal with salon waste and this may mean that some salons have different procedures to others. However, in general, hair should be incinerated, aerosols should be disposed of separately from the general salon waste and sharps should be collected by a specialist refuse company.

≫ Get up and go!

Look at the methods of waste disposal your salon adopts. How do they dispose of hair, plastics, aerosols, chemical products and sharps? Contact your Environmental Health Services department via your local authority to find out how to dispose of salon waste in the correct way. You can also ask your assessor about the different strategies in place that aim to minimise the effects on the environment of salon waste disposal. Have there been any changes or updates to best practice? Present your findings to your assessor.

Checking and cleaning equipment

All salon equipment must be checked visually before each use and cleaned after each use in readiness for the next client. Make sure equipment is cleaned thoroughly following the manufacturer's instructions. Remember to wear suitable personal protective equipment (PPE) if using chemicals or cleaning fluid. Electrical equipment should be checked by a qualified electrician and PAT (Portable Appliance Test) tested each year. This will satisfy any health and safety checks your salon has.

Floors, seating, working surfaces, mirrors and basins must also be cleaned on a daily basis using appropriate cleaning equipment. Depending on how big your salon is, you may have independent cleaners who clean on a regular basis.

Towels and gowns

To avoid cross-infection, it is very important that clean towels and gowns are used for each client. Cross-infection is when an infection (such as a cold) or an infestation (such as head lice) is passed from one person to another. Make sure you have clean gowns and towels for every treatment.

As mentioned earlier in the unit, regular checking of the day's appointments will help you plan ahead. You will need to find out how many chemical and non-chemical treatments are booked in for the day so you can ensure you have the appropriate number and colour of clean towels for each client. At the start of each day, make sure there are enough clean towels and gowns to last. This part of your work is very important – if there are not enough clean towels and gowns, your salon cannot carry out services and treatments!

? Memory jogger

1 Why is it important to dispose of salon waste safely and correctly?
2 What are your salon's waste management procedures?
3 What are sharps?
4 What does PAT stand for?
5 What needs to be cleaned in the salon every day?

» Get up and go!

Think about how it might be possible to improve the stock system at your salon. You could suggest a computerised system if the salon currently uses a manual one. If this isn't possible, why not come up with some improvements for the current system, such as using differently coloured pieces of paper to indicate how urgently ordering is needed or to list items that need ordering from different suppliers? Is this something you could discuss at one of your staff meetings?

Maintain the work area for hair services (2)

Stock

Stock is all the products, such as shampoo, conditioner, hairspray, colour, perm lotion, etc., and consumable equipment, such as hair grips, end papers, etc., that your salon needs to run smoothly. Stock-taking systems vary from salon to salon. It is your responsibility to make sure that no product falls below the minimum stock level and these levels will need to be monitored on a regular basis. The stylist or senior manager will advise you on how much stock needs to be kept for each item.

Computerised stock systems

Your salon might have a computer system which updates stock levels as you enter sales. The system may also contain other information about the salon such as clients' records and details of each stylist's income and retail sales.

Storing stock

Make sure you know how and where to store materials, tools and equipment within your salon. Your responsibilities under the current COSHH Regulations are important when handling hair products and cleaning and disinfecting/sterilising chemicals. Some items of stock will need to be stored in a locked cabinet at ground level because of the chemicals they contain, including hydrogen peroxide, straightening products, bleaching, perming and neutralising products, and certain cleaning and disinfecting materials.

Consider your salon stock room and how the stock is stored. Ideally, nothing should be stored above head height, and all heavy items, such as large containers of shampoo and conditioner, should always be stored on the floor. Everything should be tidy and easy to find. Stock rotation should be practised so that older items are used before new ones.

Be knowledgeable about the stock your salon uses. Know what each product and item is for and how it should be used properly. Use personal protective equipment as appropriate when handling, storing or disposing of certain items.

Cleaning work surfaces

Cleaning work surfaces effectively and leaving them ready for further treatments should include not just the parts of the salon used by clients, but the areas where you mix and prepare chemicals and make drinks. The floor, reception seating area, all working surfaces and mirrors must be kept hygienically clean. Any spillages on the floor must be cleared away immediately. Remember to wear personal protective equipment if necessary.

Floors will need to be swept throughout the day and mopped at the end of each day with a suitable disinfectant. Mirrors should be wiped with a suitable glass cleaner to avoid smearing and all working surfaces must be cleaned with a bactericide. To minimise cross-infection, it is essential to follow good housekeeping practices at all times.

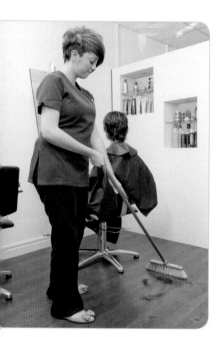

Floors will need to be swept throughout the day

Health and safety laws require salons to keep their refreshments area separate from areas where chemicals are mixed or disposed of. This is essential to good hygiene and a professional standard of working.

Getting ready for assessment

Evidence requirements

You will be observed by your assessor on at least three occasions, all of which will involve a direct observation by your assessor for three different hairdressing services.

What you must cover during your practical assessments

Performance criteria

In order to perform this unit successfully you must:

Prepare for hair services by:

- setting up materials, tools and equipment for hair services following the stylist's instructions
- making sure that materials, tools, equipment and work area are ready in time for the service
- making sure that all tools for hair services are cleaned, disinfected and or sterilised using suitable methods
- obtaining any client records in time for consultation by the stylist.

Maintain the work area for hair services by:

- disposing of hair and waste materials safely and correctly
- checking and cleaning equipment according to manufacturer's instructions and your salon's requirements
- making sure there are enough clean gowns and towels to last through the working day
- keeping stocks of products and other items needed for hair services replenished to the levels required by your salon
- storing records, materials and equipment in the required place
- cleaning work surfaces effectively, leaving the work area in a suitable condition for further services.

What you must know

In order to pass this unit you will need to gather evidence to support a consistent performance with colleagues and clients. You should also collect evidence to show that you have taken part in self development activities over a period of time. This evidence will also be signed off in your candidate handbook, which you will be given by your assessor. This will be an official record to show that you have covered what you need to.

> **? Memory jogger**
>
> 1 What types of item need to be stored in a locked cabinet?
> 2 Why is it important to regularly check stock levels?
> 3 Why should you not make a client's drink in the same area you use for mixing hair products?

UNIT GH2

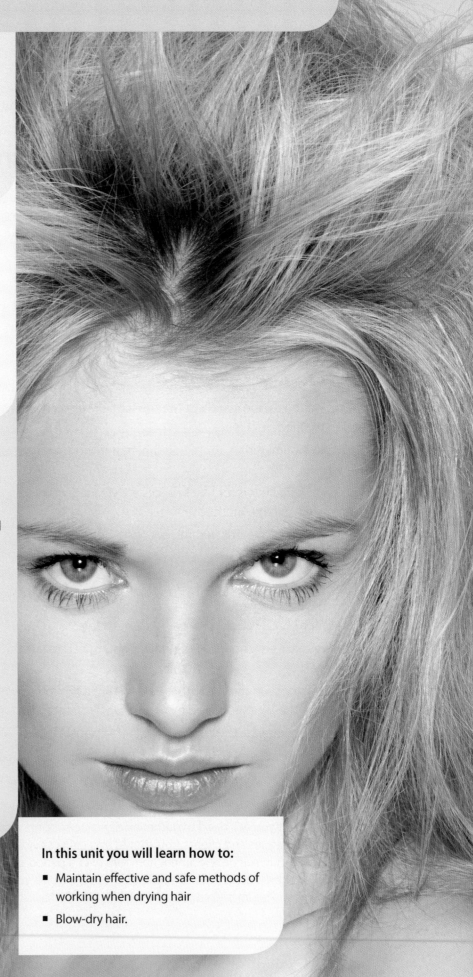

Blow-dry hair

The cut and colour of a hairstyle are of course important, but blow-drying finishes the look. A hairstyle is an expression of a person and their personality – a statement of how they feel. Your client may wear their hair simply and understated at work during the day, but then require a sophisticated or fashionable look for the evening.

A hairstyle needs to complete the overall look the client is after and a professional blow-dry can help them achieve this. It is as important as wearing the right shoes to go with an outfit! Most clients will feel more confident after having a professional blow-dry as part of their treatment, and some will come to your salon for this service alone.

This unit is about carrying out basic blow-drying techniques following the instructions of your stylist, and applies to both hairdressing and barbering salons.

In this unit you will learn how to:

- Maintain effective and safe methods of working when drying hair
- Blow-dry hair.

Here are some key terms you may meet in this unit:

Humidity –
the amount of moisture
in the atmosphere

Cross-infection –
an infection that can be passed
from one person to another

Infestation –
a large number of parasites,
e.g. an infestation of the hair
and scalp with head lice

Disinfection –
using chemicals and other
methods to reduce the
probability of infection

Sterilisation –
complete destruction of
all living organisms

Texture –
the way hair feels, determined
by touch and helps you decide if
hair is porous or non-porous

Cuticle –
outside layer of the hair shaft

Cortex –
where chemical changes take
place in the hair shaft

Medulla –
the part of the hair shaft that is
full of air spaces and which plays
no part when treating hair

Autoclave –
sterilisation system which
works under pressure
using water

Ultraviolet cabinet –
sterilisation system that
uses an ultraviolet light
to kill bacteria

Commercially viable time –
this basically means good
value for money, i.e. hair
cut = 30 mins

Maintain effective and safe methods of working when drying hair (1)

Protecting the client

As a first step when working in the salon, you must always protect your client and their clothing when preparing them for their service or treatment. The service could be a non-chemical treatment such as a blow-dry, set, hair cut or conditioning treatment, or perhaps a chemical treatment, such as a colour, bleach or perm. Make sure your client's clothing is effectively protected throughout the service and check with your stylist the most appropriate way to protect them. Many salons use the following items to protect clients:

- towels
- gowns
- waterproof capes.

Of course, all protective equipment should be clean. No one wants to smell the odour of the previous client or a previous treatment on the gown they are wearing. Clean resources also reduce the risk of **cross-infection** and **infestation**. Protective equipment should always be in plentiful supply and good condition.

> **>> Get up and go!**
>
> Start to buy the *Hairdressers Journal* and use it to put together your own style book. You can then use your style book when you are consulting with clients about how they want their hair to be styled. Remember to consider the different types of clients who may visit your salon and include styles that will appeal to them. Remember to use gents' and children's hairstyles.
>
> Look at your family's and friends' current styles – could you suggest something a little different to complement their features? Think about the practicalities of using your style book. It needs to be durable and waterproof and possibly sectioned into short, medium and long hairstyles.

Positioning your client

You will need to position your client in order to carry out the service, but you should do so without making them uncomfortable. You should also be aware of your own positioning and posture while you are working, ensuring you are minimising the risk of injury to yourself, and others. Having a good posture throughout the working day will help prevent you from feeling physically tired and, as a result, you should be able to work more efficiently.

For the blow-dry service, the client needs to be encouraged to sit square in the chair (not to one side) with their legs uncrossed. Sitting with crossed legs will lead to an unbalanced hairstyle. As the stylist, you need to stand with your feet hip-width apart and distribute your weight evenly over both legs (don't put all your weight onto one leg). Keep your head up and try to avoid stretching over the client or work area. Following these simple steps will minimise the risk of injury and fatigue.

Keeping a safe and clean work area

By keeping your work area clean and tidy throughout the service you will be able to make the best use of your time. If you regularly clear away used resources and things you no longer need, you will be able to access the things you do need easily and without delay. Making effective use of your time also means being organised and planning ahead so you're not constantly going back and forth across the salon to get equipment and products. Remember to prepare items like styling mousse, hairspray and a back mirror for finishing the service. Your client will be impressed at your professionalism and will be happy they are not kept waiting unnecessarily.

To ensure a safe working environment, all tools and equipment must be cleaned and sterilised in the correct way before being used. These measures will minimise the risk of **cross-infection** and **infestation**. Use appropriate cleaning materials to clean the areas you are working in and make sure you clean them regularly.

? Memory jogger

1 What items can be used to protect your clients?

2 For what reasons should clean protective equipment be used for each new client?

3 Why should a client be encouraged to sit with their legs uncrossed?

4 How should you position yourself when working on a seated client?

5 Why should all tools be cleaned and sterilised prior to each client?

6 How can you make effective use of your time?

Maintain effective and safe methods of working when drying hair (2)

Sterilisation methods

Moist heat

Moist heat is used in an **autoclave**, which works rather like a pressure cooker. The distilled water inside the autoclave is heated to a temperature of approximately 125°C and must only be used for small pieces of equipment which have been cleaned using hot soapy water before being put into the autoclave. The autoclave will sterilise hard rubber, such as vulcanised rubber combs, and small metal pieces of equipment such as scissors. This method will make your tools sterile which means they are completely free from all bacteria.

Liquid chemicals (barbicide)

This can be an effective method of sterilising tools, provided the tools have been cleaned with warm soapy water first. The tools must then be immersed in the liquid and left for at least one hour.

Ultraviolet light

An **ultraviolet** (UV) **cabinet** uses UV light rays to kill bacteria. Again it is only effective when the tools are cleaned beforehand with warm soapy water and allowed to dry before placing them in the U.V. cabinet. The UV light must reach all surfaces and this means you must turn your equipment in order to sterilise all sides.

Always remember to read and follow the manufacturers' instructions when using your salon's preferred method(s) of **sterilisation**.

Personal hygiene

As you are working in very close contact with clients and colleagues, you must make sure you smell clean and fresh every day. Personal clothing comes into contact with the skin and must be changed daily. You should also bathe or shower every day to remove body odour. Always use an effective deodorant on clean skin and practise good dental hygiene. Brush your teeth at least twice a day and consider using a mouth freshener such as a mouthwash. Regularly check your breath for stale smells of last night's dinner and perhaps cigarette smoke.

Your hands are in constant use and will carry bacteria from one place to another. Wash them regularly and keep your fingernails clean and free from sharp or broken edges. Cover any cuts in the skin on your hands with a suitable dressing. By having good personal standards of health and hygiene you will be minimising the risk of cross-infection, as well as giving a professional image and not offending your clients!

» Get up and go!

Take photographs in your salon or cut pictures from trade magazines of each of the following pieces of equipment: back mirror, combs, crimpers, flat brushes, handheld dryer, heated rollers, hood dryer, hot brushes, rollers, round brushes, section clips, straighteners, tongs.

Make a collage of the tools and equipment you are likely to work with every day. Perhaps you could involve a few colleagues and develop this as a small project.

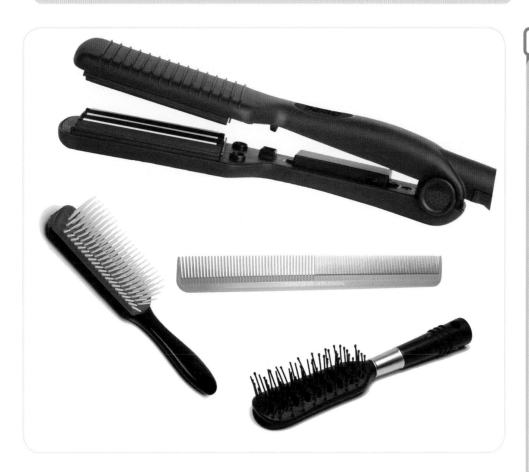

? Memory jogger

1 Name three methods of sterilising tools and equipment in the salon.

2 What is the most effective method of sterilising small pieces of equipment in the salon?

3 Before using your chosen method of sterilisation, what must you do to your tools and equipment?

4 State the common name of one infestation you are most likely to find in a hairdressing salon.

5 How can you prevent body odour and bad breath?

Blow-dry hair (1)

In order to complete this unit successfully, you must carry out blow-dry services on two different hair lengths: above and below the shoulders, creating volume and movement. Pages 144–146 show step-by-step procedures for these.

Before you carry out a blow-dry service, you should always:

- work closely with the stylist and follow their instructions
- ask questions to check you understand
- be sure there is agreement between you, the stylist and the client regarding the desired style
- check what type of products you will be using, if required at all.

If you are unsure or do not understand, always double-check with your stylist or a senior member of staff.

Observation

Watch your stylist as part of your professional development and take note of how they control their styling tools and equipment to minimise the risk of damaging the hair or causing the client discomfort. These skills must be practised many times before becoming perfect. The direction of airflow is important to achieving the desired look and avoiding damage to the hair **cuticle**.

Tools and products

The tools and products you use must be safe and fit for the purpose of hairdressing. The risk of damage to tools and equipment must be kept to an absolute minimum as they are expensive and may be made dangerous as a result. Always store your salon's equipment safely and in the correct place – this will give good value for money and ensure equipment remains in good working order.

- Make sure there are no kinks or knots in the cables of your dryer or other pieces of equipment.
- Never turn electrical equipment on or off with wet hands.
- When choosing brushes to blow-dry with, consider the **texture**, natural movement, density and length of the client's hair.
- Radial brushes create a soft rounded movement through the hair. The diameter of a radial brush will determine the size of the curl achieved on your client's hair.

- Using straighteners requires a steady hand and careful handling. Straighteners reach very high temperatures in a matter of seconds and you must know how to use them before attempting to use them on clients. They must always be used on dry hair and you should check the client's hair is in good enough condition to cope with the high temperature. For the time being, you may be able to use them on a client only under close supervision. For best results, take small sections, comb through and place the hair between the two plates. Gently close the plates and take the straighteners through the length of hair, allowing the section to drop. This will smooth the **cuticle** layer of the hair shaft and give a very professional finish to the style.

- Since working in a salon, you have probably noticed the tools of the trade are often personal to the stylist. Many stylists have favourite brushes, combs and scissors and are not always happy to share their equipment. Should you ever need to borrow a piece of equipment, be respectful by looking after it and returning it as soon as possible, clean and sterilised.

≫ Get up and go!

Draw up a list of the different styles which are achieved through blow-drying in your salon. Consider hair lengths and hair types.

Ask each stylist how long it would take to complete each blow-dry style, including any additional straightening or tonging. Compare these findings with what is considered to be an acceptable commercial timeframe.

Discuss your findings with each of the stylists. Remember, though: it is not a race, and sometimes hair density can play an important part in the length of time it takes to blow-dry a client's hair.

? Memory jogger

1 Explain why it is important to direct the airflow from a handheld dryer correctly.

2 What factors influence the choice of style you will create?

3 What should you think about when choosing a brush?

4 Why is it important to know how to use straighteners correctly?

5 List the tools you need to carry out a blow-dry.

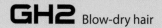

Blow-dry hair (2)

The blow-dry service

Once your client's hair has been shampooed, the style discussed and chosen, and any application of products has been agreed by both your client and stylist, you can then start to blow-dry the client's hair.

The client

Your client must always be looked after throughout the service.

- Regularly check they are comfortable.
- Make sure there isn't any water or product running down the client's face.

Technique

- The blow-dry service must be completed within a **commercially viable time** and this is usually 30–45 minutes, depending on the length, type, density and **texture** of the client's hair. Make sure your client knows how long the service will take before you start.
- Work on towel-dried hair, not dripping wet hair.
- Don't drop wet hair onto dry hair as this will make the sections you have dried flop and lose shape.
- Wet hair is more delicate than dry. Any tugging may cause hairs to break, as well as causing your client discomfort and annoyance.
- In order to prevent burning your client's skin and hair, causing hair damage or discolouring the hair, keep your dryer moving and always follow the direction of the hair shaft. This will smooth the **cuticle** layer, giving a sleek, shiny finish.
- When your client's hair is delicate, keep the dryer on a cool setting and at least 1.25 centimetres away from the hair and scalp.
- Show the client the style as you build, develop and work towards the finished look. Use the back mirror and double-check the style is going according to your client's wishes.
- Allow the hair to cool after blow-drying. Doing this fixes the style in place and prolongs the length of time the style will keep its shape. Separate the hair using your fingers or use a tail comb if needed.
- Once you have completed the blow-dry, check with your client and stylist that the style meets both their requirements.
- Apply finishing products such as serum or hairspray if required.

⟫ Get up and go!

A good hairdresser will always advise their client on ways of maintaining their hairstyle at home. What aftercare advice can you give to your clients? Think about making an 'aftercare card', perhaps the size of a credit card, which you can give to clients after a blow-dry. Make sure the tips are easy to read and keep the information brief. You could include something like:

- Towel dry hair before blow-drying.
- Comb hair from the ends.
- Keep the hairdryer moving all the time.
- Avoid excessive heat.
- Minimise the use of straighteners.
- Remember to protect your hair from the sun.
- Avoid using rubber bands to hold your hair up.
- Use serum on dry hair to protect it.

⬆ Get ahead

Look back at the different face shapes on page 100. What styles would you suggest for each?

? Memory jogger

1 Why should you always advise the client how long a blow-dry will take?

2 Why should you take care to keep wet hair away from pre-dried hair?

3 Why should sections of hair be kept damp before blow-drying?

4 When giving a blow-drying service, when should you show the client their hair in the back mirror?

5 What are the benefits of allowing hair to cool before dressing out?

6 Why is it important to give your client aftercare advice?

Blow-dry hair (3)

Blow-drying using a radial brush

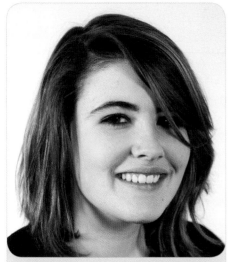

1   Correctly gown the client and, after your consultation, take them to the basin for shampooing and conditioning

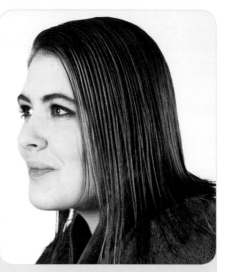

2   After rinsing, towel dry the client's hair and comb through before you begin to section

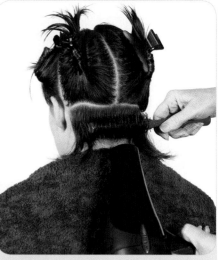

3   Place the brush horizontally into the section of hair and take through to the ends, wrapping the ends around the brush. Follow through with the dryer and dry from the roots to points

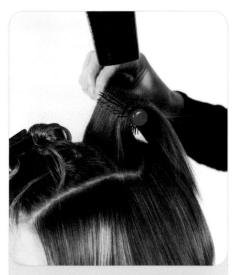

4   To encourage root lift, lift sections straight up from the crown. Check with your client if the style is developing as required

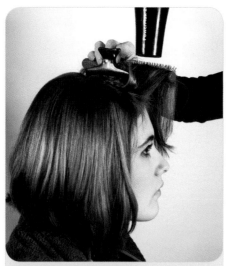

5   Position yourself parallel to the section you are working on and complete the front section

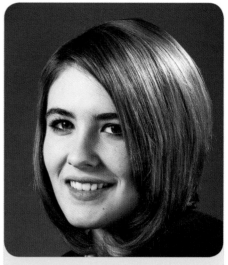

6   Apply products such as spray or serum to complete the look as required

Blow-dry hair (4)

Blow-drying using a flat-backed brush

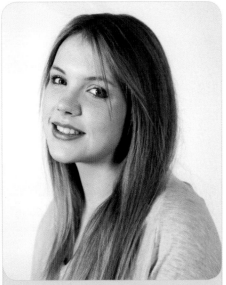

1 Correctly gown the client and, after your consultation, take them to the basin for shampooing and conditioning

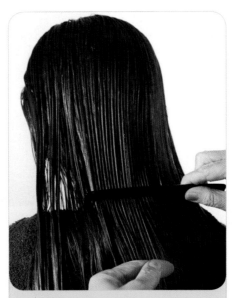

2 After rinsing, towel dry the client's hair and comb through before you begin to section

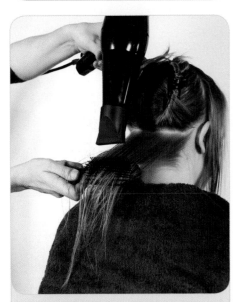

3 Place the flat brush under the roots of the hair and blow dry, encouraging root lift and volume. Keep the dry hair from falling onto wet hair

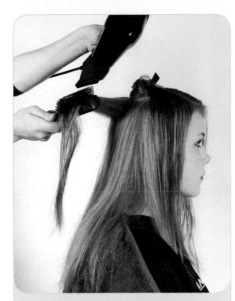

4 Continue to move through the blow dry from the nape to the occipital bone, remembering to incorporate the sides of the client's head

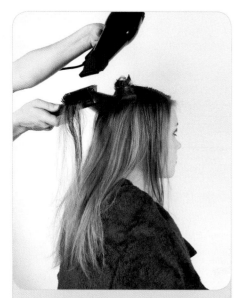

5   To encourage a smooth and shiny look, direct the dryer down the hairshaft

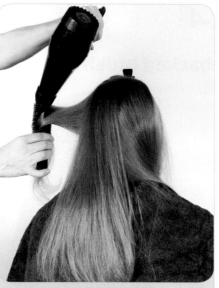

6   You should stand parallel to the section you are blow-drying when incorporating the sides. Check with the client if they are happy with the style as it develops

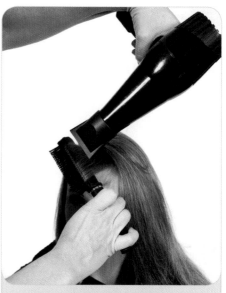

7   Angle the dryer and brush to finish the fringe area

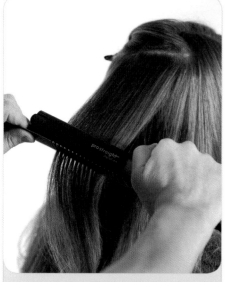

8   Use straighteners and a comb for a polished finish

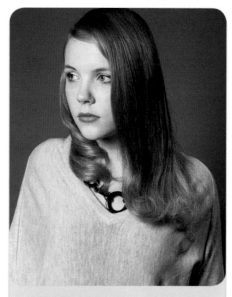

9   The finished look – apply products such as spray or serum to complete the look as required

Getting ready for assessment

Evidence requirements

You will be observed by your assessor on at least three occasions, this must involve all blow-drying techniques, all hair lengths and all types of tools on three different clients. This unit also includes an external paper.

What you must cover during your practical assessments

Ranges

In this unit you must have covered the ranges below:

- tools for blow-drying
- above and below shoulder length hair
- blow-drying covers.

Performance criteria

In order to perform this unit successfully you must:

- maintain effective and safe methods of working when blow-drying hair.

Blow-dry hair by:

- confirming instructions with the stylist prior to starting the service
- applying products if required
- controlling tools and equipment to minimise risk of damage to the hair and client discomfort
- checking your client is comfortable during the drying process
- using your tools and equipment to achieve the required result
- effectively controlling your client's hair during the blow-drying process
- drying hair to meet your stylist's instructions.

What you must know

In order to pass this unit, you will need to gather evidence to support a consistent performance with colleagues and clients. You should also collect evidence to show that you have taken part in self development activities over a period of time. This evidence will also be signed off in your candidate handbook, which you will be given by your assessor. This will be an official record to show that you have covered what you need to.

UNIT GH4

Assist with hair colouring services

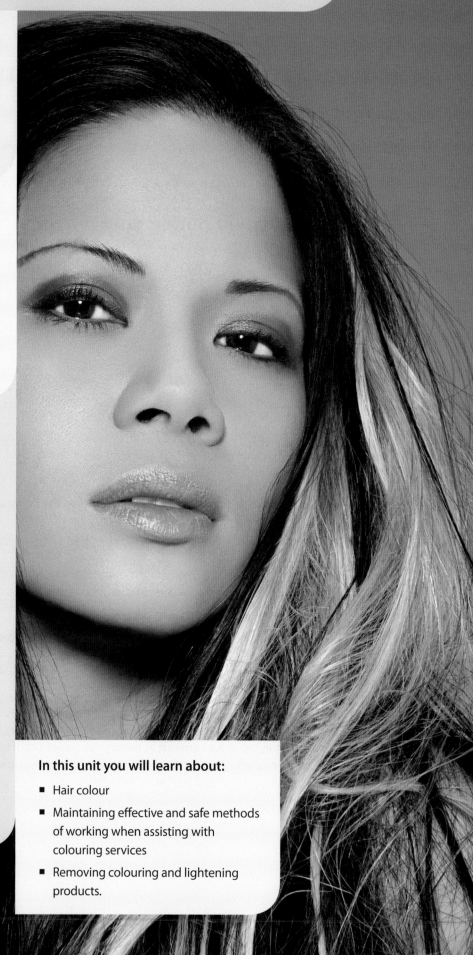

Not everyone is happy with their natural hair colour. Some of your clients may feel that their natural colour doesn't suit them, they have too much grey or that their style may look more up to date with a colour change. With the help of their salon, it is now possible for clients to achieve a natural looking hair colour change – or not so natural, if they want an unusual colour! Colouring hair can also add depth and shine, as well as lift the natural hair colour and leave it in better condition than before. Your clients do not even have to commit to a permanent colour, so can change their mind later and try something completely different.

This unit is about the basic skills of removing colouring and lightening products. The work involved will be carried out under the direction of the relevant person such as the stylist or assessor. This unit applies to hairdressing students working in hairdressing and barbering salons.

In this unit you will learn about:

- Hair colour
- Maintaining effective and safe methods of working when assisting with colouring services
- Removing colouring and lightening products.

Here are some key words you may meet in this unit:

Dermis –
the inner layer of the skin

Eumelanin –
brown/black pigment
in the hair

Pigment –
a substance that colours
tissue, such as hair and skin

Pheomelanin –
red/yellow pigment in the hair

Cortex –
layer of the hair where
chemical changes take place

Surface conditioner –
conditioner which coats the
outer layer of the hair shaft

Cuticle –
outer layer of the hair shaft

Tangle-free –
hair which has been combed
smooth and is free from
knots or tugs

Antioxidant conditioner –
conditioner which penetrates
into the cortex layer of the
hair shaft

Minimise –
reduce the effect
of something

Fatigued –
exhaustion from over work or
adopting a poor posture

Emulsify –
using the colouring product to
help remove itself by moving
the finger pads around the
client's hairline

Hair colour

What gives hair its natural colour?

Hair colour is genetic, which means the natural colour of your hair is a result of the mixture of both your mum's and your dad's genes. You do, however, usually receive a predominant gene for hair colour from either your mum or your dad, e.g. your mum or dad might have a strong red pigment as their natural colour. This colour may then dominate your natural colouring.

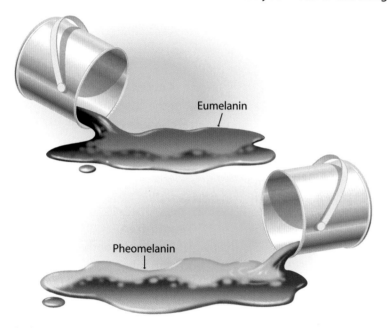

When we look more closely at the process of how hair develops beneath the skin, we can see how hair colour cells produce colour. Cells called melanocytes in the cortex of the hair shaft produce two colour pigments called:

- **eumelanin**
- **pheomelanin.**

Everyone has varying proportions of eumelanin and pheomelanin. People who have naturally brown or black hair will have lots of the pigment eumelanin. People who have red or blonde hair will have more of the pigment pheomelanin.

Which pigment have you got more of: eumelanin or pheomelanin?

> **» Get up and go!**
>
> Gather together some paints in primary colours (red, yellow and blue). Mix together in equal quantities:
>
> - red and blue
> - red and yellow
> - yellow and blue.
>
> What new colours did you create? You should have created purple, orange and green. These are secondary colours. By changing the amounts of each primary colour you mix together, you can create your very own colour. Which colours complement each other and go together well? Which ones don't go so well together? Be creative and make decisions about the colours you are making and mixing. Colouring hair can be creative and fun, and you can apply some of the skills you have just learned when in the salon.

Shades of hair colour

Colours come in different shades, which is how light or dark they are. When you look at a hair shade chart you will notice there is a numbering system. Hair shades are numbered between one and ten, with ten being the lightest (blonde) and one being the darkest (black).

Black, brown, red or blonde?

As we have already learned, hair colour comes from the **pigments** produced in the hair shaft. Different combinations of these pigments produce the many different natural colours and shades of hair. If a person has no pigments in the hair shaft, he or she will have white hair – this is due to the melanocytes no longer producing colour pigment. Reasons for white hair include ageing, heredity, trauma, shock, stress or childbirth. Interestingly, redheads have more hair than brunettes, and brunettes have more hair than blondes.

Colouring hair in the salon

Chemical treatments such as hair colouring and lightening may be offered in your salon. A new hair colour can completely change a client's look. Some of your clients may have experimented with colouring at home, which can be fun and done in no time at all. However, a professional colouring service carried out at a salon can give a much better result, with the added benefit of an expert opinion on what colour to go for.

Your salon may stock the following colouring products:

- temporary colours
- semi-permanent colours
- quasi-colours
- permanent colours
- lightening products
- vegetable colours.

The rest of this unit will deal with working effectively and safely when assisting with colouring services. You will also learn about removing colouring and lightening products from the hair, and materials such as foils, Easi Meche and the highlighting cap.

> **» Get up and go!**
>
> Test some hair samples with different types of colour. Note down the differences in hair condition and the colour result achieved. Perhaps you can make up your own shade chart.

> **? Memory jogger**
>
> 1 Name the two pigments found in hair colour.
>   Which gives black/brown hair? Which gives blonde/red hair?
> 2 What happens if a hair contains no pigment?
> 3 How do hair shade charts work?

Maintain effective and safe methods of working when assisting with colouring services (1)

Protecting the client

When preparing a client for a colouring service, or any other service, you must make sure they are properly protected. Use clean towels, gowns and waterproof capes. Follow the instructions of the stylist; they will tell you how best to protect the client, and may ask you to use specific towels for chemical treatments such as colouring.

Don't forget to take care of the client by offering them a drink and a magazine. The best time to do this is probably when the chemical treatment is processing.

Preparing the client for shampooing

Before shampooing, you will need to comb through the client's hair. Remove tangles carefully to avoid causing the client any discomfort. Check the client's scalp with the stylist, looking for any cuts or areas of irritation that may need special attention. You will also need to discuss with the stylist the correct shampoo to use.

> **» Get up and go!**
>
> Does your salon have a towel system? Find out if they do and, if so, what colour towels are used for different treatments. For example, what towel would you use for a permanent colour? What colour towel would you use for a bleach treatment?
>
> Salons use a lot of towels each day. Encourage your salon to go green, if it isn't already. This means washing towels on a cool or warm water programme. The electricity bill will be lower and the salon's energy usage will be more efficient, which is better for the environment.

Personal protective equipment (PPE)

You must always remember to wear personal protective equipment (PPE) when working with clients who are receiving a chemical treatment. Your hands and clothing must be protected at all times. Dermatitis is caused by an irritant coming into contact with the skin and can make skin dry, itchy and sore. Use barrier cream or a good quality hand cream when working in the salon to help prevent your skin from drying out. Protect your skin completely by wearing gloves when applying colouring products, rinsing colours and using hydrogen peroxide or bleaching products.

Positioning the client and checking your own posture

As you are preparing the client for shampooing, ask whether they would prefer a front-wash or back-wash basin if a choice is available. Position the client at the basin and make sure they are comfortable. Make sure the client's neck is positioned correctly in the curve of the basin, otherwise the nape area may not be shampooed properly. By thinking about your own posture and standing correctly while shampooing you can reduce the risk of injury and **fatigue**. It is also a good idea to offer the client a towel to safeguard against unavoidable splashes.

Keeping your work area clean and tidy

It is essential to keep your work area clean and tidy during chemical treatments. Think about the tools, equipment and products you are going to need and make sure you have them to hand. Clear away anything that has been used and won't be needed again. This will ensure you don't waste time or keep your client waiting while you go back and forth getting things, or look for the things you need in a messy work area. Keeping your work area clean and tidy will enable you to work more effectively and it also helps keep your workplace safe.

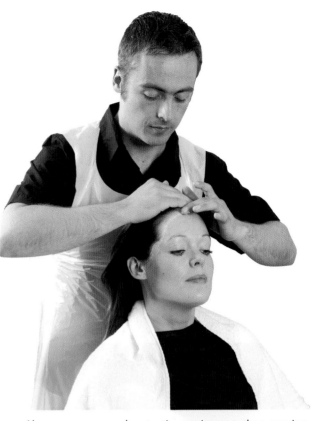

Always wear personal protective equipment when carrying out a chemical treatment

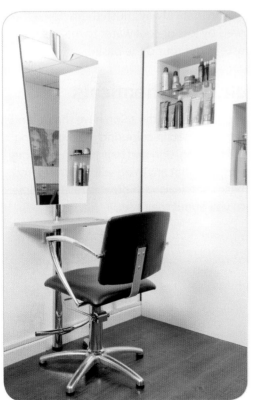

The work area should be kept clean and tidy

? Memory jogger

1 What should always be done before shampooing the client?

2 What does PPE stand for? Give some examples of PPE, along with when and why they should be used.

3 What is dermatitis and what causes it? How can you prevent it?

4 Why might you use a front-wash basin?

5 How would a dirty and untidy work area affect your work?

Maintain effective and safe methods of working when assisting with colouring services (2)

Reducing product wastage

Before using chemicals, always read the manufacturer's instructions and discuss them with the stylist. If you are asked to mix a chemical product, remember to mix only the amount you need just before it is to be used. Some manufacturers advise using scales to weigh the product, or you may use a measuring beaker instead in order to achieve an accurate mixture. Taking these steps will help to reduce product wastage. If extra product is required, it is more cost-effective to make it freshly as it is needed.

Disposal of chemicals

It is very important that you dispose of chemicals in the proper manner. Your salon must follow the Control of Substances Hazardous to Health (COSHH) Regulations (see page 20) and ensure products are disposed of in a safe and environmentally friendly way. Some salons have a specific basin for disposing of chemicals. Never pour chemicals down the sink in the salon's food and drink preparation area. Always flush them down the shampoo basin, followed by lots of cool water to make sure no smells or chemical waste linger round the basin.

Working safely with chemicals

Some of the products you will use in the salon have the potential to cause harm. The chemicals used in colouring and lightening treatments can damage clothing, skin and hair. However, if they are used correctly it is unlikely that anything will go wrong. You must always handle these chemicals with great care and follow all instructions given to you about their use.

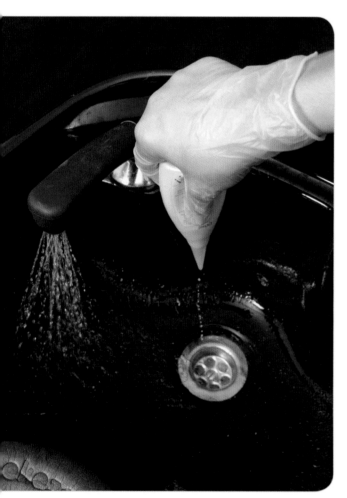

Chemical waste should be flushed down the shampoo basin

You can reduce the amount of contact a chemical has with the client's skin by using barrier cream around the hairline. You should also always check you are using the right type of heat with each product or you could cause the client to suffer from chemical burns. If you ever have any concerns or problems, it is best to check with the stylist or assessor promptly and find out the correct course of action to take.

Re-ordering products

If the stock levels of a product are running low, remember to follow your salon's policy for re-ordering, which will probably involve telling the appropriate member of staff or writing it down. This will ensure you have sufficient products available, and also avoid having too much stock.

> **» Get up and go!**
>
> With a colleague, find out:
> - the different types of colouring and lightening products available in your salon
> - how they are applied
> - how long they last on the hair.

Reducing the risk of harm or injury to yourself, your colleagues and clients

Always keep a look out for hazards or risks which may arise during the course of the day. Clear away used product bottles and used materials such as bowls and cotton wool. Keep the floor clear from trailing cables, towels, gowns and cut hair, as well as items belonging to clients such as handbags, shopping bags, walking sticks and pushchairs. This will help to **minimise** the risk of any accidents occurring.

? Memory jogger

1 Why wouldn't you mix up all the chemicals you need for the day's appointments at the start of the day?

2 What might happen as a result of pouring chemicals down the basin used for washing up and preparing drinks?

3 How would you use barrier cream to protect your client?

4 How can you reduce the risks of accidents in your salon?

Maintain effective and safe methods of working when assisting with colouring services (3)

Reducing the risk of cross-infection

Cross-infection is when an infection is passed from one person to another. You can take some very simple steps as you work to reduce the risk of this happening. Remember to always practise good personal hygiene and wear clean, well-pressed clothes. If you or any of your clients are showing signs of infection or infestation, you must report it straight away to a senior member of staff. They can then advise you what to do. You should also make sure you know how to use your salon's methods of sterilisation properly and ensure you always use clean tools and equipment on each new client.

It is not just for reasons of hygiene that tools and equipment should be properly cleaned. Cleanliness can also make the difference between achieving a professional result and a poor result from colouring and lightening. Make sure brushes and mixing bowls are always washed free of product so as not to contaminate the next product they will be used with. You should also have a different brush for each product you are applying. For example, do not mix bleach with a tint brush that has been used for applying a raspberry grape tint!

 Salon life

In error, you use a tint brush for bleaching which was used previously to apply a rich red colour, but had not been washed out properly. What would happen to the client's hair colour?

Skin tests

Client preparation for colouring and lightening treatments varies from salon to salon, but it is very likely a skin test will need to be carried out 24–48 hours before the service can take place. This will ensure it is safe for the treatment to go ahead and the client won't suffer from any reaction to the product when it is applied. Skin tests will almost certainly be required for most semi-permanent colours, quasi-colours and permanent colours, but may also be needed for vegetable colours too. You must follow the instructions you are given for skin tests very carefully or the consequences could be serious. The results must be recorded on the client's record card.

If your client has sensitive skin or has reacted to other products, natural products such as vegetable colours can sometimes be safer alternatives. They are unlikely to cause dermatitis and do not usually require a skin test. Remember, though, not all clients can use natural products on their skin, so it is still worth checking the suitability first. The processing of vegetable colours may require exposure to oxygen in the atmosphere, which means the final colour result will not be achieved until the day after the treatment.

Incompatibility tests

Another type of test that may be carried out is an incompatibility test. This is where the stylist makes sure the client's hair is able to be coloured or lightened. Previous treatments or hair in poor condition can cause undesirable results. For example, metallic salts which are found in hair colour restorers and compound henna may cause the hair to boil, bubble and break during lightening treatments. If metallic salts are suspected, the stylist will not proceed. As with skin tests, the results should always be noted on the client's record card.

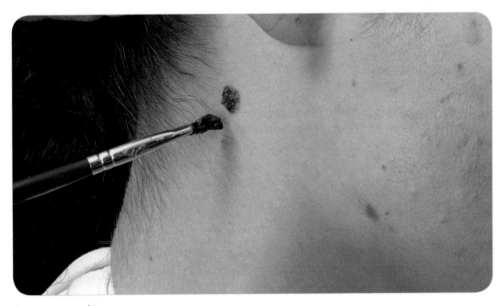

Carrying out a skin test

? Memory jogger

1 What can you do to reduce the risk of cross-infection?

2 How soon before a colouring or lightening treatment should a skin test be carried out?

3 Are vegetable colours always safe to use on everyone?

4 Why is an incompatibility test carried out?

5 Where should the results of any test be recorded?

≫ Get up and go!

With the help of a stylist, carry out an incompatibility test. You will need:

- a sample of hair
- a non-metallic bowl
- hydrogen peroxide
- perm lotion.

Ask your stylist about other types of hair and scalp tests, such as porosity tests and elasticity tests.

Removing colouring and lightening products [1]

Resources for colouring and lightening

You will need to prepare a trolley for the stylist with the following items:

- client record card
- clean towels (of the appropriate colours)
- barrier cream
- cotton wool
- shade chart
- foils or Easi Meche
- highlighting cap and hook
- tinting bowl and brush
- hydrogen peroxide (sometimes).

» Get up and go!

With a colleague, practise setting up a trolley for a colour or lightening treatment. Check each other's trolleys for any missing items. Now set up a trolley for each other, but deliberately forget one item. See if you can spot what is missing.

Assisting with the colouring process

Your role in the colouring process includes preparing the client for the treatment and removing any materials (such as foils, a highlighting cap or Easi Meche) and products from the hair after the treatment.

Always check with the stylist before removing colouring or lightening products and materials and follow the manufacturer's instructions. You must learn to remove products and materials in a way which minimises the risk of damage to the hair and colour being spread to the client's skin, clothing and surrounding areas of hair. Some colouring and lightening products require you to **emulsify** them before water is applied to the hair and scalp. This is important as the colour will not come off the skin if you miss this simple step.

Should there be any problems, refer them to the relevant person, usually the stylist, who will advise you what to do. The types of problems you may come across include the following.

- Colour bleeding onto an area of hair that has not been coloured.
- Bleach splashing into a client's eyes.
- Ripped hair, caused by the highlighting cap being removed roughly.
- An unsatisfactory result, which can be caused by Easi Meche or foils being removed before the end of the processing time.

The table below shows some common colouring problems and how to deal with them.

Fault	By whom	Correction	How to avoid
Colour seepage	Stylist	Recolour areas as necessary	Apply barrier cream to the areas not being coloured
Bleach in client's eyes	Stylist	Rinse with cool water immediately	Careful removal of colouring materials and products
Vigorous removal of the highlighting cap	Junior	Condition hair and massage scalp	Apply conditioner to the top of the cap before removing
Hair colour too warm	Stylist	Apply toner	Check base shade and use correct strength of products

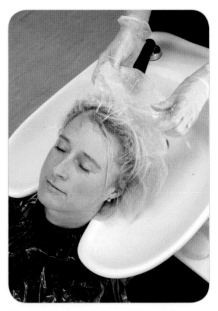

To remove a highlighting cap, apply some anti-oxy conditioner and gently ease the cap from the client's head, checking that there is no discomfort

1 Protect the client with a towel, gown and waterproof cape

2 Prepare the client for colouring with the stylist. This involves hair and scalp analysis, and combing and sectioning dry hair

3 After the stylist has applied the colour and it has been allowed to process, remove the colouring products

4 Rinse the hair

The colouring process

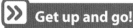
Removing colouring and lightening products (2)

Applying conditioner

Once you have removed all of the colouring or lightening product, you may have to use a colour removal shampoo. Following this, squeeze out excess moisture from the hair then apply a suitable **antioxidant conditioner** or **surface conditioner**. Antioxidant conditioners will need to be left on the hair for at least three minutes. Antioxidant conditioners will:

- replace lost moisture
- help prevent further oxidation of the hair
- return the pH of the hair to its normal acid value.

Ask your stylist which conditioner to use.

Preparing the client for the next treatment

After rinsing the conditioner from the client's hair, towel-dry the hair and scalp and make sure they are free from excess products and moisture. Help the client to the styling area and comb the hair through, leaving it **tangle-free** without damaging the hair or scalp. Both the stylist and client need to be satisfied that you have removed all traces of product from the client's hair. Should you have any concerns about the products or how to use them, promptly refer any problems to your stylist or assessor for the appropriate course of action.

Remember to clean and tidy the basin area after you have prepared the client for the next treatment. Make sure all used products are disposed of correctly and leave the area free from risks of hazard, cross-infection or infestation, ready to be used by the next client.

After-colour care

It is important to explain to clients how they should look after their hair at home. After-colour care involves helping the client to maintain the colour of his or her hair at home using the most appropriate shampoo and conditioner for colour-treated hair. This is part of professional client care, and by selling the client the correct products, you will be giving him or her expert advice and guidance which completes the colouring treatment.

? Memory jogger

1 Colour has run into your client's eyes. What course of action would you take?
2 Name three things antioxidant conditioner does.
3 What are the benefits of offering clients aftercare?

Get ahead

This book contains a number of step by steps, which show how some practical hairdressing tasks are carried out. Have a go at creating your own step by step showing how to apply semi-permanent colour. Take photographs in your salon and then arrange the photos in order so someone could follow the process. You might want to use the following steps as a guide to taking your photos.

- Step 1: The equipment you will need.
- Step 2: Shampooing the client.
- Step 3: Sectioning the hair into four.
- Step 4: Applying the product to the back of the head using either a tint brush and bowl or applicator bottle.
- Step 5: Applying the product to the side of the head.
- Step 6: Applying the product to the top of the head.
- Step 7: Working the product into the hair shaft.
- Step 8: Leaving the colour to process as per the manufacturer's instructions.
- Step 9: Shampooing and rinsing the product off.
- Step 10: The finished dried and styled result.

Perhaps you could display your step by step photos in your salon to help your junior colleagues. You could even create step by steps for other treatments.

Getting ready for assessment

Evidence requirements

You will be observed by your assessor on at least two occasions, one observation must involve the removal of colouring materials. This unit also includes an external paper.

What you must cover during your practical assessments

Range

In this unit you must have covered the range below:

- different types of colouring product.

Performance criteria

In order to perform this unit successfully you must:

- maintain effective and safe methods of working when assisting with colouring services
- remove colouring and lightening products using appropriate techniques and products to minimise the risk of damage to the hair.

What you must know

In order to pass this unit, you will need to gather evidence to support a consistent performance with colleagues and clients. You should also collect evidence to show that you have taken part in self development activities over a period of time. This evidence will also be signed off in your candidate handbook, which you will be given by your assessor. This will be an official record to show that you have covered what you need to.

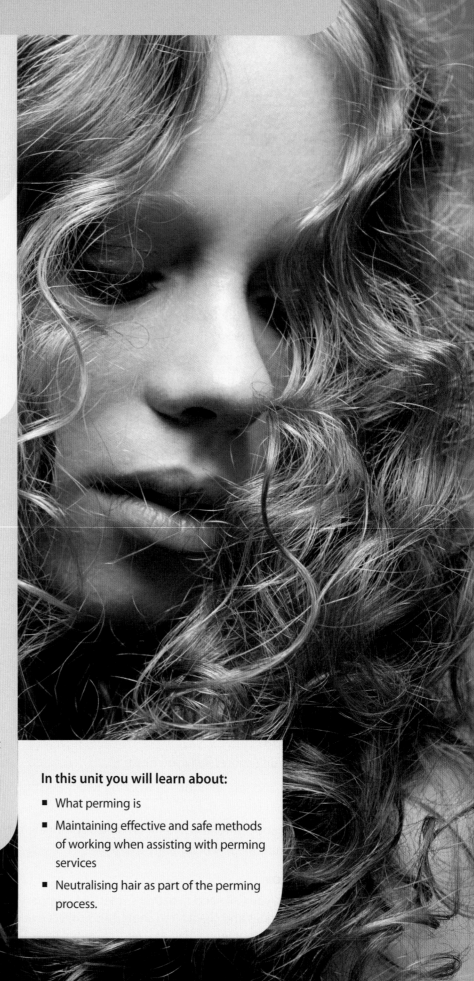

UNIT GH5

Assist with perming hair services

The reason some people have straight hair and others have curly hair is down to the shape of the hair shaft. A naturally straight hair has a circular cross-section, whilst a naturally curly hair has an oval cross-section. It is now understood that the hair follicle also has a big part to play in determining the curliness of hair as it affects the shape of the hair shaft, as well as the angle it grows at. In order to make straight hair curly, as happens during a perm, hairdressers have to change the structure of the hair using chemicals. This is now a safe process and can achieve incredible results.

The work involved in this unit should be carried out under the direction of the relevant person, such as the stylist or assessor. This unit will apply to hairdressing students working in both hairdressing and barbering salons, and is suitable for those working with Caucasian and Asian hair types.

In this unit you will learn about:

- What perming is
- Maintaining effective and safe methods of working when assisting with perming services
- Neutralising hair as part of the perming process.

Here are some key terms you may meet in this unit:

Cortex –
layer of the hair where chemical changes take place

Cuticle –
outer layer of the hair shaft

Disulphide bonds –
keratin bonds which are linked together in the cortex

Asian hair –
the hair shaft is round in shape, straight and/or coarse

Surface conditioner –
conditioner which coats the outer layer of the hair shaft

Tangle-free –
hair which has been combed smooth and is free from knots or tugs

Texture –
the way hair feels, determined by touch during the consultation

Neutralising –
the process that fixes hair into its new shape

Fatigue –
exhaustion from over work or adopting a poor posture

Perming –
curling hair by using a chemical product

Caucasian hair –
the hair shaft is oval in shape and can be straight, wavy or curly

Anti-Oxy conditioner –
conditioner which penetrates into the cortex layer of the hair shaft

What is perming?

The desire to have curly hair is an old one and throughout history women, in particular, have tried various methods to transform their limp, straight hair into a bouncing head of curls. Hair can be made curly by simply wetting it and winding it, as well as through the use of heated styling equipment. These results are only temporary though and often don't achieve the desired look. With a permanent wave (or perm) curls can be chemically added to straight hair, although straight hair will grow back from the roots.

> **»** **Get up and go!**
>
> List the different ways in which curls or waves can be added to hair without the use of a perm. Discuss these with your stylist, considering the pros and cons of each.

Perms work by using chemicals to cause a permanent change in the structure of keratin, the protein found in hair. There are two main stages to **perming** hair.

- Stage 1: A chemical is added to the hair that breaks open the **disulphide bonds**, which give hair its elasticity, in the **cortex** layer of the hair. This stage must be carefully timed to ensure the correct amount of bonds are broken.

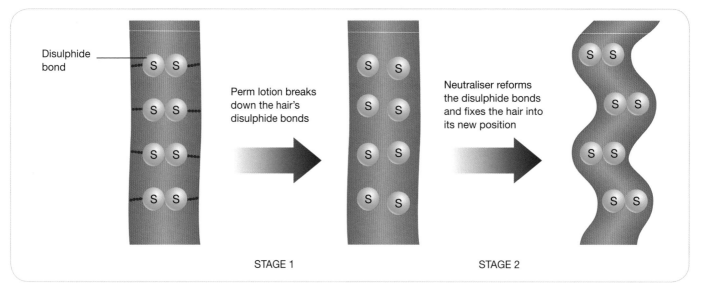

Disulphide bond

Perm lotion breaks down the hair's disulphide bonds

Neutraliser reforms the disulphide bonds and fixes the hair into its new position

STAGE 1

STAGE 2

The two stages of perming

- Stage 2: A second chemical containing hydrogen peroxide or sodium bromate is used to close the bonds, which causes the hair to take on the shape of the rods. This is called **neutralising**. Again, timing is essential when completing this stage in order to achieve the desired result and not damage the hair.

Because the change caused by **perming** is permanent, it can only be removed by cutting or growing the hair out, or reversing the treatment chemically.

Acid and alkaline perms

Perms can be of the acid or alkaline variety. Alkaline perms contain ammonia and have a pH of between 8.2 and 9.6. Acid perms have a pH of between 4.5 and 6.5 (remember, hair is acidic with a pH of between 4.5 and 5.5). Alkaline perms work more quickly than acid perms and usually hold their shape for longer. Acid perms act more slowly and are gentler on the hair. A stylist will choose either an acid or alkaline perm depending on the result required and the client's hair type and condition. Hair which is dry, damaged or porous will be better suited to an acid perm, which is less likely to cause damage.

Considering hair types when perming

Chemical treatments for **Caucasian** and **Asian hair** types are slightly different and you will need to be able to work with both. The differences between Caucasian/European and Asian/Oriental hair are important when choosing the most appropriate product. The Caucasian/European hair shaft can be straight, wavy or curly and has an oval cross-section. The Asian hair shaft can be straight and/or coarse and is round in shape.

The texture of hair will vary from client to client and may also vary within the same head of hair. Texture can be fine, medium or coarse, with fine hair having a small circumference and coarse hair a large circumference. To determine the texture, run your fingers along the length of a single hair. This information will be useful when you are choosing products.

>> **Get up and go!**

What types of perm lotion are used in your salon for different hair types and conditions? Discuss them with your senior stylist.

? **Memory jogger**

1 Describe the two stages in perming hair.

2 Why might an acid perm be more suitable for some clients' hair?

3 Explain the difference between Caucasian/European hair and Asian/Oriental hair.

4 How can you determine the texture of hair?

Maintain effective and safe methods of working when assisting with perming services [1]

Salon life

Why might a salon use different coloured towels for perming and neutralising?

Protecting the client

Make sure your client is suitably protected for the perming service. Use clean gowns, towels and waterproof capes. Your salon may use specific towels for chemical treatments and different ones for non-chemical treatments.

Personal protective equipment (PPE)

Remember to wear personal protective equipment (PPE) when working with clients who are receiving a chemical treatment. Your hands and clothing must be protected at all times. Wear gloves when rinsing perm lotion and neutralising products from the hair. This is to protect yourself from the damage that perming chemicals can potentially cause.

Preparing the client for shampooing

Before shampooing, you will need to comb through the client's hair. Remove tangles carefully to avoid causing the client any discomfort and check the client's scalp with the stylist for any cuts or irritated areas. You will also need to discuss with the stylist the correct shampoo to use.

The pre-perm shampoo

The pre-perm shampoo will remove any build-up of hair-care products, open the cuticles and leave the hair at a neutral pH of 7 ready for either an acid or alkaline perm lotion.

Positioning the client and checking your own posture

Ask the client if they would prefer a back-wash or a front-wash basin if available and position them carefully, checking they are comfortable. Remember to think about your own posture during the shampoo so as to reduce the risk of injury or fatigue.

Preparing the resources for perming

You will need to prepare a trolley for the stylist with the following items:

- client record card
- clean towels (of the appropriate colours)
- barrier cream
- cotton wool
- gloves

- apron
- a selection of combs
- plastic bowl
- plastic cap*
- rods

- section clips
- tension strips
- Climazone or other heat source*

- gown
- waterproof cape
- end papers.

* These items may be needed

All resources must be cleaned or sterilised after every use. This will help to minimise the risk of cross-infection.

Familiarising yourself with manufacturers' instructions

Here is a typical list of manufacturers' perming instructions.

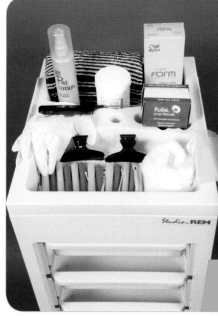

A trolley prepared for perming

Vitality

Vita Perm

Permanent wave

Instructions for use (read thoroughly).

1 Preparation:
- Check the condition and porosity of the hair then select the correct lotion.
- Shampoo the hair using a mild shampoo. Rinse thoroughly and towel-dry.
- To equalise hair porosity for an even curl result, a pre-perm treatment is recommended.
- Section the hair and select appropriate curler size for the chosen technique, then wind without lotion. Vitality End Papers make winding easier.

2 Application:
- Wear protective gloves.
- Carefully apply the perm lotion onto each curler, using the applicator nozzle.
- Repeat if necessary to ensure thorough penetration, but do not over-saturate.
- Allow to develop.

3 Development guidelines:
The suggested development times in the guidelines overleaf have been tested thoroughly and produce optimum results. However, if you are unsure about the overall condition and porosity of the hair, we recommend test curls should be taken to determine the final development time. Development times can be increased as required but care should be taken to avoid over-processing. When correct curl strength is achieved, rinse hair thoroughly for five minutes.

4 Rinsing and neutralising:
After completion of development time rinse all curlers thoroughly (2–3 minutes). Thoroughly blot the curlers to remove excess moisture.

Foam neutraliser:

- Pour 50ml of the neutraliser into a non-metallic bowl.
- Add an equal amount of warm water. The neutraliser is now ready to use.
- For maximum neutralisation, use a neutraliser sponge and apply two thirds of the neutraliser evenly to all the curlers, foam up thoroughly (do not foam up in the bowl).
- Leave to develop for five minutes.
- Gently unwind all the curlers and apply the remaining one third of the neutraliser through the hair.
- Distribute evenly and allow to develop for a further five minutes.
- Rinse thoroughly.
- Blot out excess moisture with a clean towel.

5 After care:
After rinsing out we recommend the use of a suitable after-care treatment.

Vitality UK Ltd. Newtown NW1 1AB

Maintain effective and safe methods of working when assisting with perming services (2)

Assisting with the perming service

1 Ensure the trolley is prepared prior to perming

2 Protect the client with towels, a gown and a cape

3 Carry out a hair, skin and scalp analysis by dividing the hair into sections

4 Pass rods and papers to the stylist as they need them

Keeping your work area clean and tidy

Look at page 153 in Unit GH4 to find out how you can keep your work area clean and tidy, and why this is important.

Reducing product wastage

Look at page 154 in Unit GH4 to find out how you can limit the amount of products your salon wastes.

> **» Get up and go!**
>
> You could try to interest clients in perming services by wearing your own hair curly. Try curling your hair a couple of times during the week and take notice of the comments your clients make. Talk to them about the advantages of curling their hair and show them suitable styles.

> **» Get up and go!**
>
> Find out how to prepare a neutraliser your salon uses by reading the manufacturer's instructions. Discuss the result, and how you found following the instructions, with a senior colleague.

Disposal of chemicals

Look at page 154 in Unit GH4 to find out how to properly dispose of chemicals in the salon.

Reducing the risk of harm or injury to yourself, your colleagues and clients

Look at page 155 in Unit GH4 to find out how you can reduce the risk of harm or injury to yourself, your colleagues and clients.

Reducing the risk of cross-infection

Look at page 156 in Unit GH4 to find out what cross-infection is and how you can take some simple measures to reduce the risk of it happening.

Skin and incompatibility tests

Skin tests involve applying a small amount of a product to the client's skin in order to ensure it is safe for a chemical treatment such as **perming** to go ahead. The test usually needs to be carried out 24–48 hours before the service can take place. You must follow the instructions you are given for skin tests very carefully or the consequences could be serious.

An incompatibility test involves taking a sample of the client's hair and applying the product to it. This is to make sure the client's hair is in a suitable condition to cope with the chemical treatment. The result of any test must be recorded on the client's record card.

Tests must be carried out in accordance with manufacturers' instructions and recognised industry practices.

> ### ≫ Get up and go!
>
> Ask your stylist about other types of hair and scalp tests that are carried out, such as pre-perm test curl, development tests, porosity tests and elasticity tests.

> ### ≫ Get up and go!
>
> With a colleague, find out:
> - the different types of perming products available in your salon
> - how they are applied
> - how long they last on the hair.

> ### ? Memory jogger
>
> 1 How would a dirty and untidy work area affect your work?
> 2 Why wouldn't you mix up all the chemicals you need for the day's appointments at the start of the day?
> 3 How can you reduce the risk of accidents in your salon?
> 4 What might happen as a result of pouring chemicals down the basin used for washing up and preparing drinks?
> 5 What can you do to reduce the risk of cross-infection?
> 6 Where should the results of any test be recorded?

Neutralising hair as part of the perming process [1]

Rinsing out the perm lotion

You will need to follow both the stylist's and the manufacturer's instructions when rinsing the client's hair free of perm lotion. At the end of the processing time, the hair should be rinsed for a minimum of five minutes to thoroughly remove all traces of perm lotion. It is best to use warm water, which will leave the **cuticles** of the hair open, enabling the neutraliser to penetrate more effectively.

Towel-blotting the hair

The hair must be free from excess water before the neutraliser is applied. To remove excess moisture, you will need to towel-blot the hair. It is worth taking time to do this properly as too much water in the hair will dilute the neutraliser and ruin the perm. Check how wet the hair is by placing your hands over the rods – if you find lots of water on your hands, you must continue with towel-blotting. Some salons may use tissue or cotton wool to remove excess water from the client's hair.

Applying the neutraliser

As you have already learned, neutraliser closes the bonds that were broken by the **perming** lotion and fixes the hair into the shape of the rod being used. There are two main types of neutraliser used in the salon:

- hydrogen peroxide neutralisers
- sodium bromate neutralisers.

Correct timing of the **neutralising** process is crucial to the finished result. Over-processing can leave the hair frizzy, and under-processing will give a weak curl result. Make sure the client's skin is well protected before applying the neutraliser. Use barrier cream and damp cotton wool around the hairline.

You must match the neutraliser with the perm lotion being used. For example, an alkaline perm must be followed through with a hydrogen peroxide neutraliser. Some neutralising products can be used straight from the bottle, whilst others will need foaming up in a bowl first. The stylist will instruct you on how to use a particular product. You should also read the manufacturer's instructions, which will explain how to use the neutraliser safely and effectively.

Make sure you apply the neutraliser evenly throughout the client's wound hair, taking care to avoid any area which has not been permed. Unpermed hair can be protected by applying gel or conditioner. Leave the neutraliser on the client's hair for the recommended length of time. This will ensure the **disulphide bonds** are fixed into their new position. You may find it helpful to use a timer to accurately time the processing. Some types and lengths of hair may need a longer time to develop depending on the amount of hair wound around the rod.

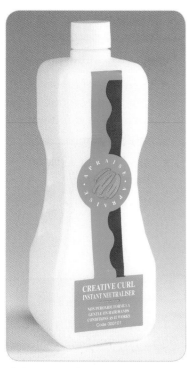

An example of a neutralising product

? Memory jogger

1 How long do you rinse the client's hair prior to applying neutraliser?

2 Why towel-blot the hair before applying neutraliser?

3 Name the two types of neutraliser.

4 Why is timing the neutralising process correctly so important?

≫ Get up and go!

Discuss with your assessor the reasons why you would not massage or rub the scalp vigorously when rinsing out chemical products.

1 Position the client at the basin and rinse hair thoroughly

2 Towel-blot the hair to remove excess water

3 Check there is no excess water by pressing your hands over the rods

4 Apply the neutraliser to each rod and allow it to process according to the manufacturer's instructions

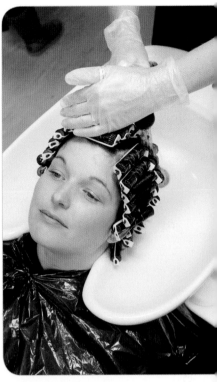

Neutralising hair as part of the perming process (2)

Rinse the perm for at least 5 minutes

Removing the rods

With some neutralisers you will need to leave the rods in place during processing. Others require you to remove the rods after five minutes before continuing with the second part of the process. Always check the instructions to make sure you are using the product correctly. When you do remove the rods, you will have to do so very carefully so as not to disturb the curl and cause the hair to become straight. The hair is also in a very delicate state at this time and any rough handling can cause irritation to the client's scalp. Check with your stylist whether or not you should apply more neutraliser.

Removing the neutraliser

After the neutraliser has been left to process for the appropriate time, rinse it off thoroughly so that no traces are left in the hair. This will prevent chemical damage to the hair and makes sure the new shape is fixed.

Applying conditioner

Remove excess moisture from the client's hair by squeezing out the water by hand. Then apply a suitable **antioxidant conditioner** to the client's hair. Leave the conditioner on the hair for at least three minutes and then remove it, rinsing thoroughly. Towel-dry the client's hair and wrap it in a turban style before showing the client to the styling area. Comb through the hair, leaving it tangle-free for the next treatment. Make sure you leave the basin area clean and tidy ready for the next client.

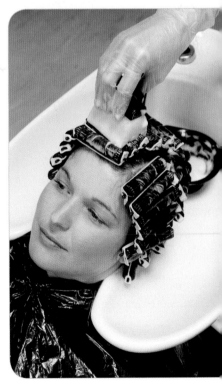

Applying neutraliser

Perming and neutralising problems

Perming and **neutralising** problems might include the hair returning to its natural straight look if the neutraliser is left in too long, frizziness, uneven curls along the hair length, straight hair at the sides or nape, or an irritable scalp. Mistakes can and do happen in the salon. When they do, stay calm and refer to the senior stylist immediately. To minimise the risk of a problem occurring, make sure you listen to all instructions given to you and check the manufacturer's instructions for each product.

The table opposite shows some common perming problems and how to deal with them.

Fault	By whom	Correction	How to avoid
Fish hooks	Stylist	Remove by cutting	Cover points of hair with end papers
Over-processing	Stylist/Junior	Cut and condition	Carefully time the process using the salon clock or a timer. Record the processing time on the record card
Neutraliser applied unevenly	Stylist/Junior	Re-perm if the condition of hair allows	Check the stylist's/manufacturer's instructions. Monitor application of neutraliser
Skin and scalp irritation	Junior	Rinse immediately with cool water	Carry out appropriate test before chemical treatment
Hair breakage	Stylist	Cut to disguise and use restructurant to strengthen hair	Carry out incompatibility test and pre-perm treatment

> **» Get up and go!**
>
> Not all product manufacturers produce a post-perm treatment. Some offer a product which can be used across a range of perms. Find out what products you can safely use for which perms. Discuss this with your assessor.

After-perm care

It is important to explain to clients how they should look after their hair at home. After-perm care involves helping the client to maintain their perm at home using the most appropriate shampoo, conditioner and styling products for permed hair. This is part of professional client care, and by selling the client the correct products, you will be giving him or her expert advice and guidance which completes the **perming** treatment.

Get ahead

Working either with a colleague or a training head, practise winding a spiral perm. This method of perming is time-consuming and needs you to be confident during the winding process as the sections of hair must be evenly wound around the bendy spiral rod. The hair you work on should be medium to long, towel-dried and in neat workable sections secured with butterfly clips. Start by taking sections of hair from the nape area, working from left to right on section one, alternating each section as you work up the client's head. This method of winding will give a degree of width on one-length hair cuts and a softer look on layered hair. Spiral perms do not promote root lift so be sure to discuss this with your client. You should aim to complete a medium-length spiral wind in one hour.

Memory jogger

1 Why do you need to remove rods very carefully?

2 Why does neutraliser need to be removed completely from the hair?

3 What are fish hooks and how are they avoided?

4 What does after-perm care mean?

Getting ready for assessment

Evidence requirements

You will be observed by your assessor on at least two occasions. This unit also includes an external paper.

What you must cover during your practical assessments

Performance criteria

In order to perform this unit successfully you must:

- Maintain effective and safe methods of working when assisting with perming services
- Neutralise hair as part of the perming process.

What you must know

In order to pass this unit, you will need to gather evidence to support a consistent performance with colleagues and clients. You should also collect evidence to show that you have taken part in self development activities over a period of time. This evidence will also be signed off in your candidate handbook, which you will be given by your assessor. This will be an official record to show that you have covered what you need to.

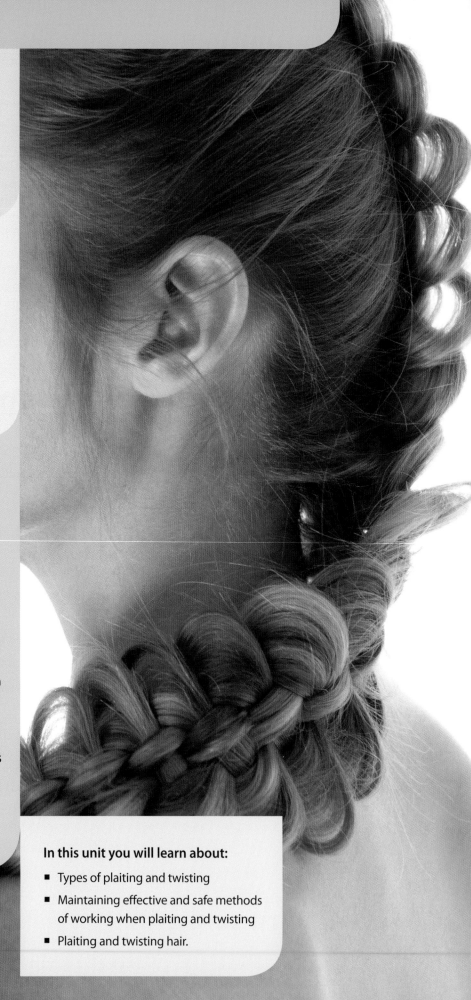

UNIT GH6

Plait and twist hair using basic techniques

Plaiting and twisting hair is a very skillful technique and requires a high degree of manual dexterity (being good at using your hands). A single plait can give either an innocent or sophisticated look, depending on the style, whilst twists can be edgy and dramatic, completely changing the client's look. Both plaiting and twisting techniques can offer your clients something a little different, whether for everyday wear or a glamorous evening look. The techniques require patience and practice to perfect but you will then be able to offer them in addition to classic salon services, such as chemical treatments, cutting and styling.

This unit is about using basic plaiting and twisting techniques following the instructions of the stylist and is suitable for those working with Caucasian and Asian hair types. This unit applies to hairdressing students working in hairdressing and barbering salons.

In this unit you will learn about:

- Types of plaiting and twisting
- Maintaining effective and safe methods of working when plaiting and twisting
- Plaiting and twisting hair.

Here are some key terms you may meet in this unit:

Sprays –
used to hold a style

Gels –
used to keep hair in place and add shine

Tangle-free –
hair which has been combed smooth and is free from knots or tugs

French plait –
usually one main plait secured to the scalp

Multiple corn rows –
lots of tiny scalp plaits

Caucasian hair –
the hair shaft is oval in shape and can be straight, wavy or curly

Asian hair –
the hair shaft is round in shape, straight and/or coarse

Serums –
oil-based products used to smooth the cuticle

Traction alopecia –
excessive tension applied to the hair and scalp causing baldness

Texture –
the way hair feels, determined by touch during the consultation

Two-strand twists –
tiny twists involving two strands of hair

Types of plaiting and twisting

Plaits are formed by intertwining (weaving together) strands of hair to create patterns or even structures. Material other than hair, such as ribbons or hair extensions, can be incorporated into the plait to give a more interesting finished look. Twists are formed by twisting sections of hair around each other. Both plaiting and twisting can create very artistic, intricate and ornate hairstyles, involving techniques that are very specialised and take time to master.

Plaits and twists can be created on short, medium and long hair, on any hair type or **texture** and on both males and females. They can be small or large and formed either close to the scalp or in loose hanging sections, giving the hair movement.

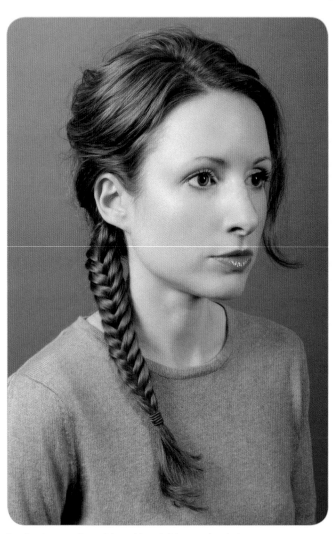 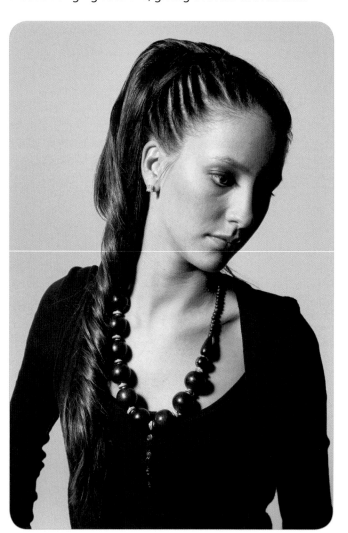

Looks that can be achieved by plaiting and twisting

Before you can proceed with a plaiting or twisting service you will need to be sure the client's hair can cope with the tension (pulling) that will be applied. You will also need to consider what styles are likely to suit them by looking at their hair and facial characteristics. You will therefore need to think about the following:

- hair type
- hair length
- hair density
- hair elasticity
- head and face shape.

Always follow the instructions of your stylist.

 Get up and go!

Get together with a colleague and think about how each other's hair type, length, density and elasticity, as well as face and head shape, will affect a plaiting or twisiting service. What style would each of you recommend to the other?

Considering hair types when plaiting and twisting

You will need to think about the type of hair your client has when carrying out plaiting and twisting techniques. **Caucasian**/European and **Asian**/Oriental hair types have important differences and you will need to be able to work with both. One of the major differences is **texture**, which will vary from client to client and may also vary within the same head of hair. Texture can be fine, medium or coarse, with fine hair having a small circumference and coarse hair having a large circumference. To determine the texture, run your fingers along the length of a single hair.

You also need to know about the dangers of applying too much pressure on the hair when plaiting and twisting. Hair that is excessively pulled can lead to a painful and irritable scalp, as well as hair breakage. If this pulling, or tension, continues the client may suffer from what is known as '**traction alopecia**', where the hair is pulled from the scalp due to excessive tension, leaving a bald area. This area will remain bald until new hair grows back through – it can be a month before you see only 1.25 cm of new hair.

 Get up and go!

Find out about the different types of equipment that are used to create plaited and twisted styles. Don't forget about things like coloured hair pieces and hair ornaments that can be added.

? **Memory jogger**

1 What types of things should you consider before carrying out a plaiting or twisting service?

2 How can Caucasian/ European and Asian/ Oriental hair differ?

3 What are the potential consequences of excessive tension on the hair and scalp?

Maintaining effective and safe methods of working when plaiting and twisting (1)

Protecting the client

Your client must be protected with clean towels, gown and waterproof cape. If your client is having colour added to their hair as part of the plaiting or twisting service, you may need to use particular towels intended for colouring. Remember that it is very important your client's clothes are adequately covered and protected during a colouring service.

Personal protective equipment (PPE)

Remember to wear suitable PPE when carrying out a plaiting or twisting service, particularly if you are using coloured **sprays** or **gels**. Gloves will protect your hands from these irritants, which can cause dermatitis.

Preparing the client for shampooing

Your client may need to have their hair shampooed before the plaiting or twisting service can be carried out. This may be due to a build up of styling products or perhaps the client's hair is excessively oily. Before shampooing, you will need to comb through the client's hair. Remove tangles carefully to avoid causing the client any discomfort. Check the client's scalp with the stylist, looking for any cuts or irritated areas which may need special attention. You will also need to discuss with the stylist the correct shampoo to use, which may be a clarifying shampoo that removes all previous products and leaves the hair in its most natural state.

Positioning the client and checking your own posture

As you prepare the client for the plaiting or twisting service, ask them whether or not they will need to move from the chair for any reason. The service may take an hour or two and so it is a good idea to find out if they have any physical needs you should be aware of. If they do need to get up and stretch or walk about during the service, you may like to offer them the opportunity to do so before you start any particularly tricky parts. Remember also to offer the client refreshments or a magazine before and regularly during the service.

As you will be working on the client for a long time, it is important to be aware of your own comfort. You should stand with straight legs and your feet slightly apart to maintain your balance. Keep your shoulders relaxed too. Taking these simple steps will help minimise your risk of developing injury and fatigue.

>> Get up and go!

What products does your salon offer that can be used to add colour to your client's hair as part of a plaited or twisted style? Should they be used on wet hair or dry hair? Do they require any processing time? Discuss your findings with your assessor.

Get up and go!

Think about the concerns usually experienced by clients when they have their hair plaited or twisted. What might they be worried about? How can you reassure them? Talk through your thoughts with your assessor.

Keeping your work area clean and tidy

It is essential that you keep your work area clean and tidy during the service. This will ensure the service runs smoothly and also gives a professional image to the client. Position tools and equipment for ease of use and prepare the trolley with all of the resources you will need for plaiting or twisting, ensuring they are clean and in good condition.

Preparing the resources for plaiting and twisting

You will need to prepare a trolley with the following items:

- client record card
- clean towels (of the appropriate colours)
- gloves
- apron
- selection of combs
- old hairdressing scissors
- extension hair (if required)
- soft bristled brush
- section clips
- aftercare products
- aftercare sheet/card.

All resources must be cleaned or sterilised after every use. This will help to minimise the risk of cross-infection.

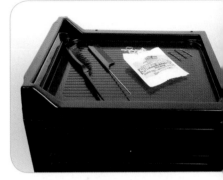

A trolley prepared for plaiting and twisting

Get up and go!

You could try to interest clients in plaiting or twisting services by trying them out on your own hair. Try wearing a couple of different plaits and twists in your hair for a few weeks and take notice of the comments your clients make. Talk to them about the advantages of wearing plaits and twists in their hair and show them some suitable styles.

? Memory jogger

1 What type of personal protective equipment is available for you and your clients?

2 Why might a client need a shampoo before a plaiting or twisting service?

3 How can your posture reduce fatigue and the risk of injury?

Maintaining effective and safe methods of working when plaiting and twisting (2)

Minimise the risk of damage to tools

The hairdressing profession relies on good quality, safe tools and equipment in good working order. Always do your best to look after your own tools and equipment and the salon's property. Before using, make sure items are safe and fit for their purpose, reporting any faults to the appropriate person.

Reducing product wastage

Before using any product, always read the manufacturer's instructions and discuss the instructions with the stylist. If you need to prepare a product, remember to prepare only the amount you need just before it is to be used. This will help to reduce wastage. If extra product is required, it is more cost-effective to make it freshly as you need it.

Reducing the risk of cross-infection

Reduce the risk of cross-infection by being alert to any signs of infection and covering any open wounds or cuts with a suitable waterproof dressing. Report any personal infection or infestation to the appropriate member of staff. Always practise good standards of personal hygiene and wear clean, well-pressed clothes every day. Clients who have an open cut or wound must be treated with particular care. Seek advice from the stylist or your assessor and find out if barrier cream would be appropriate on this occasion. The situation may require your client to return for the service once the open wound has healed.

All tools and equipment used during the service must be cleaned in the appropriate way. Make sure you are familiar with how to clean or sterilise everything you have used, including brushes, combs, section clips, gowns and towels. This will reduce the risk of cross-infection and ensure tools and equipment are kept in good condition.

>> **Get up and go!**

Discuss with a colleague what a commercially acceptable time frame for plaiting and twisting hair is. Are these services listed on your salon price list? How much do they cost? Does your salon sell any products associated with plaiting and twisting? If so, what are they, how are they applied and how long do they last?

Reducing the risk of harm or injury to yourself, your colleagues and clients

Always keep a look out for hazards or risks which may arise during the course of the day. Clear away used product bottles and used materials such as bowls and cotton wool. Keep the floor clear from trailing cables, towels, gowns and cut hair, as well as items belonging to clients such as handbags, shopping bags, walking sticks and pushchairs. This will help to minimise the risk of any accidents occurring.

Removing plaits or twists

Depending on what style your client has gone for, they may need to come back to the salon to have their plaits or twists professionally removed. They may want to do it themselves, but inform them that it can be very time-consuming. You should discuss with the client a suitable time frame to come back to the salon for a check-up appointment, which could be, say, two months after the plaits or twists were put in. Remember, the removal process must be costed as part of the salon's services and should appear on the price list. You should aim to remove a complete set of plaits or twists from short to medium-length hair in less than one hour.

? **Memory jogger**

1 What should you do if you find that a tool or piece of equipment is broken?

2 Why is it more cost-effective to make up products as you need them?

3 What might happen if the salon is left to become cluttered with used resources and items belonging to clients?

Plaiting and twisting hair (1)

Plaiting techniques – French plait

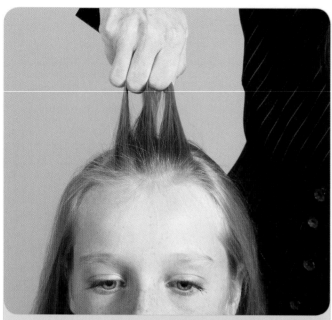

1   Correctly gown the client. Take the first section across the front hairline and divide into three strands

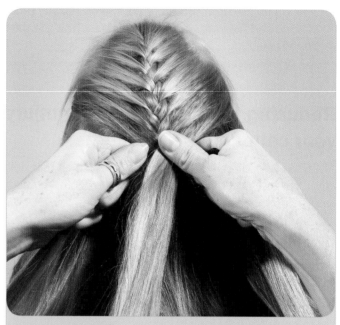

2   Cross the right-hand section over into the centre, then cross the left-hand section into the centre

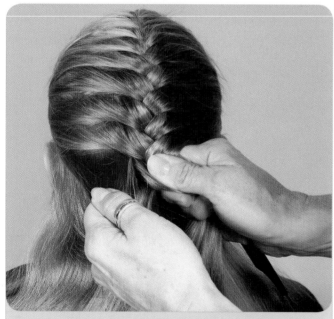

3   Pick up more hair from the sides as you work along the top of the head, keeping the hair taut. Smooth each section as you work from the front hairline section

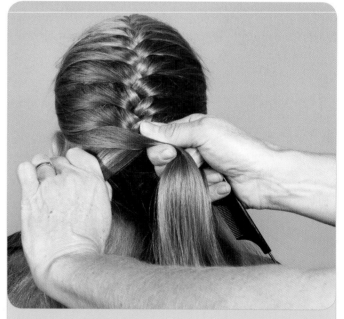

4   Keep the hair close to the client's scalp and the tension even as you continue to work towards the crown

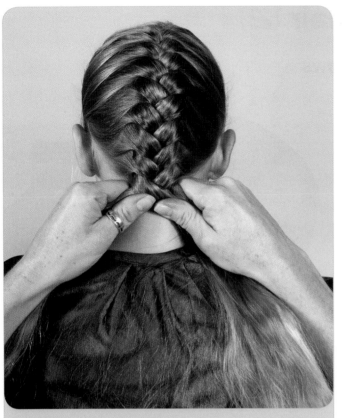

5 Continue to plait down the hair length and secure the free ends with a covered band or ribbon

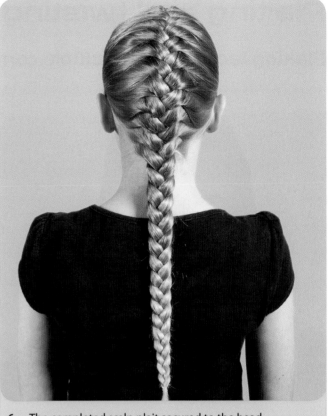

6 The completed scalp plait secured to the head

Best practice for plaiting and twisting

- Always think about your client's comfort. Are they coping with any discomfort? Do you need to stop and reduce the tension?

- Neat sections and partings are crucial to the success of a style created by plaiting and twisting. They will also increase the lifespan of the hairstyle.

- Another important factor is even tension. You will have to reach a balance between applying enough tension to create the style and not causing your client too much discomfort or even hair breakage. You will soon learn to adjust the tension of plaits or twists to suit both the style and the client.

- Sections of hair not being worked on need to be held out of the way. Use section clips or butterfly clips and bring down only the amount of hair you need to work on.

- Apply suitable products as necessary during the service, taking care to follow manufacturers' and the stylist's instructions. The types of product you may need include **sprays**, **serums** and **gels**, which will help maintain the life of the hairstyle and give a professional finish.

Salon life

List the different ways in which you can secure the client's hair when you have finished plaiting or twisting it.

? Memory jogger

1 How do you secure the hair not being worked?

2 What will help make for a successful head of twists and plaiting?

3 How often should you check the client's comfort?

Plaiting and twisting hair (2)

Plaiting techniques – Multiple corn rows

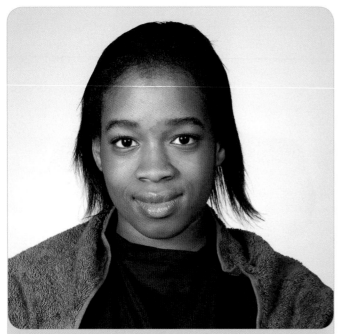

1   Correctly gown your client and, after your consultation, begin to section the hair

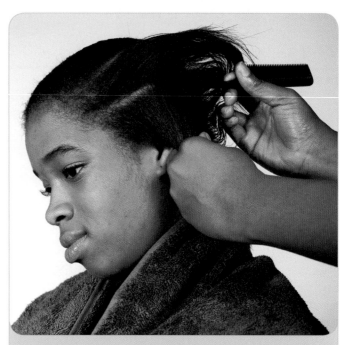

2   Begin sectioning at the sides

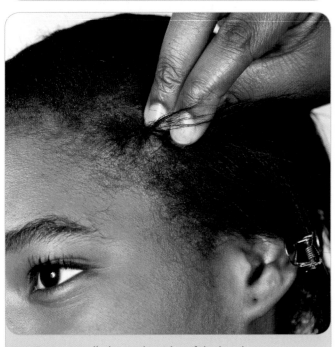

3   Form a small plait at the sides of the head

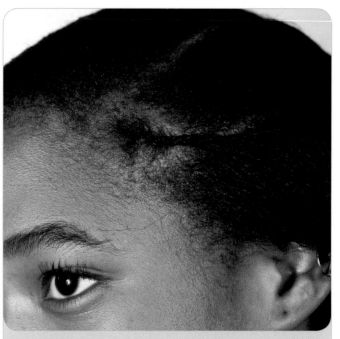

4   Work from the front hairline towards the nape area forming small neat plaits

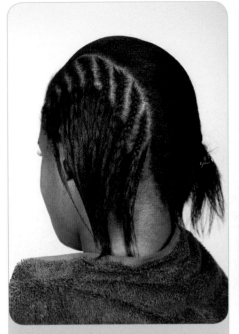

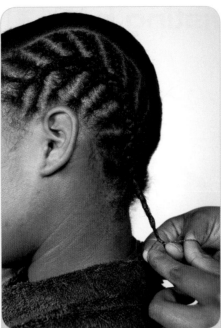

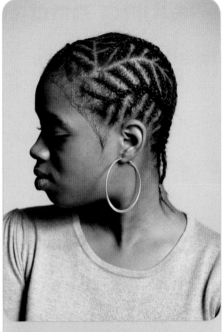

5   Plait the longer lengths together, working from the front through to the napes

6   The completed corn rows seen from the side

7   The finished look

Traction alopecia

Excessive tension (pulling) on the hair may lead to traction alopecia where the hair comes away from the scalp leaving bald areas. You will need to be alert for signs of this during a plaiting or twisting service. Look for:

- a sore/sensitive scalp
- weeping/pus at the roots
- a reduced amount of hair in an area.

Should traction alopecia occur, the area should be looked after with great care as any open sores may lead to an infection. Wearing plaits and twists continuously or regularly can lead to traction alopecia and so is not recommended. If your client becomes concerned, they should return to the salon for professional removal of the plaits or twists.

Any sign of alopecia needs to be recorded on your client's record card, noting the location of affected areas. Talk to your client about why this has happened and speak to your stylist about advice you can give to help improve the condition of their scalp.

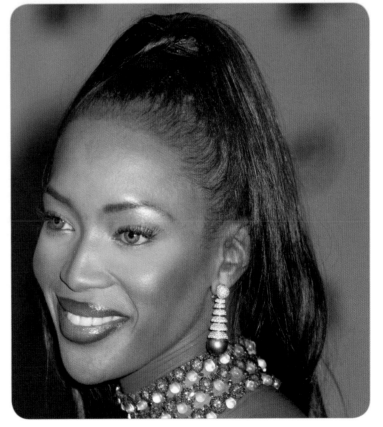

Traction alopecia

Plaiting and twisting hair (3)

Twisting techniques

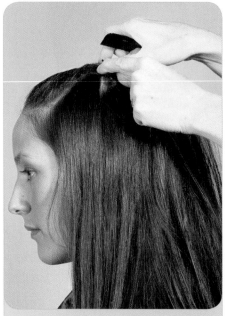

1   Prepare the client for the twisting service and begin to section the hair

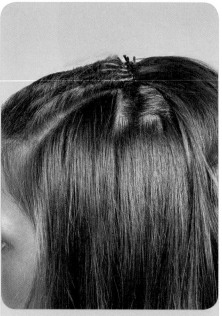

2   Take five sections and twist the hair from the front hairline working back towards the crown

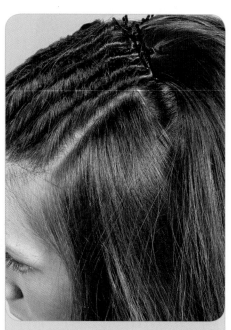

3   Secure the sections with hair grips as you work

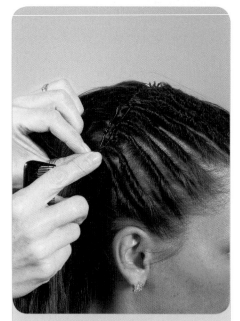

4   Work down either side starting at the top of the client's head until you reach the finished look

Aftercare

You can start to advise your client on how to look after their plaits or twists as soon as you start the service. If it is a style that is meant to be worn for more than a day or two, you should advise your client how to keep their hair clean. Shampooing is still possible but they should not rub their hair vigorously, and plaits should be washed in the direction of the plait. Suitable oils and moisturisers can also be applied to the hair in order to protect it and add shine. These measures should minimise tangles and prolong the style.

You will need to advise the client how long they can wear their hair in plaits or twists before they should have them removed so as to prevent **traction alopecia**. Finally, be knowledgeable about the retail products in your salon and give the client helpful advice about the most appropriate products for their hair and style. Aftercare is part of professional client care and completes the plaiting or twisting service.

Getting ready for assessment

Evidence requirements

You will be observed by your assessor on at least three occasions, which must include corn rows, plaits and two strand twists using all types of products. This unit also includes an external paper.

What you must cover during your practical assessments

Ranges

In this unit you must have covered the ranges below:

1 products
2 plaits and twists.

Performance criteria

In order to perform this unit successfully you must:

- Maintain effective and safe methods of working when plaiting and twisting.

Plait and twist hair by:

- preparing your client's hair and ensuring the finished plait or twist meets the stylist's instructions
- controlling your tools to minimise risk of damage to the hair and scalp, reduce client discomfort and to achieve the desired look
- effectively secure your client's hair, when necessary.

What you must know

In order to pass this unit, you will need to gather evidence to support a consistent performance with colleagues and clients. You should also collect evidence to show that you have taken part in self development activities over a period of time. This evidence will also be signed off in your candidate handbook, which you will be given by your assessor. This will be an official record to show that you have covered what you need to.

 Get ahead

Aftercare is a very important part of any hairdressing service. Clients who are well looked after are more likely to return to your salon rather than go somewhere else. Create an aftercare sheet or card for clients who have received a plaiting or twisting service. Remember to include basic details such as the salon's name and contact details, as well as your name and some advice on how they can look after their hairstyle at home. You could make this information into a list of 'dos and don'ts', for example.

? Memory jogger

1 How often should the client return for a consultation?

2 How soon do you start to advise your client on how to care for their new hairstyle?

3 Is it possible to shampoo hair with hair extensions?

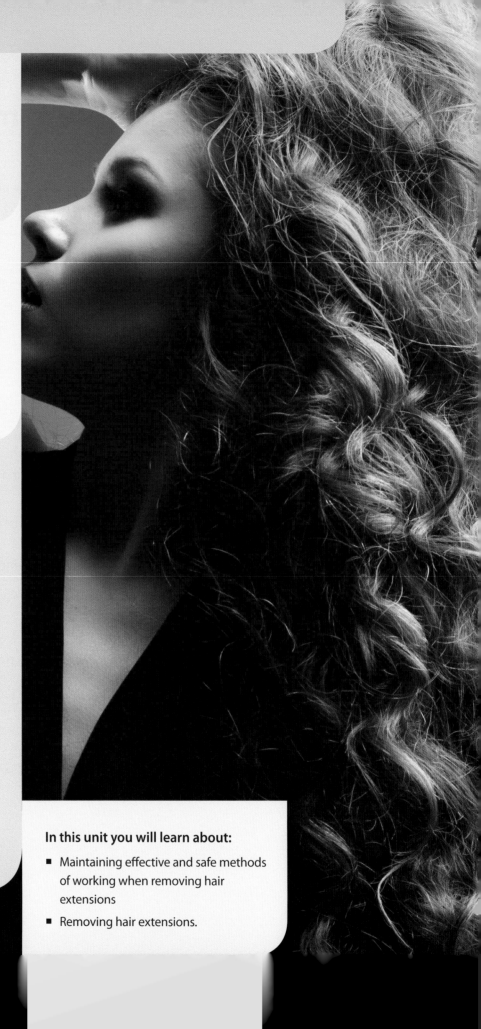

UNIT GH7

Remove hair extensions

Hair extensions can completely transform a client's look: short hair can be replaced by long flowing locks, and volume, texture, colour and curls can be added in no time at all. Hair extensions can be funky and wild or serious and sophisticated. They can be added for fun and fashion or to help a client regain their hairstyle because of thinning hair. With an increasing demand for hair extensions it is very beneficial to be able to offer your clients this service in your salon.

In this unit, you will learn how to remove hair extensions following the instructions of a stylist. You will need to be able to use a number of tools and products in order to do this effectively and safely. The work involved will be carried out under the supervision of the relevant person, such as the stylist or assessor. This unit applies to hairdressing students working in hairdressing and barbering salons and is suitable for those working with Caucasian and Asian hair types.

In this unit you will learn about:

- Maintaining effective and safe methods of working when removing hair extensions
- Removing hair extensions.

Here are some key terms you may meet in this unit:

Tension –
pressure applied to the hair and scalp by excessive pulling

Seal breaker –
implement used to assist with removal of hair extensions

Traction alopecia –
excessive tension applied to the hair and scalp causing baldness

Asian hair –
the hair shaft is round in shape, straight and/or coarse

Caucasian hair –
the hair shaft is oval in shape and can be straight, wavy or curly

Extensions –
additional hair applied to natural hair to offer length, texture, volume and colour

Cuticle –
outer layer of the hair shaft

Surface conditioner –
conditioner which coats the outer layer of the hair shaft

Tangle-free –
hair which has been combed smooth and is free from knots or tugs

Fatigue –
exhaustion from over work or adopting a poor posture

Texture –
the way hair feels, determined by touch during the consultation

Maintaining effective and safe methods of working when using hair extensions (1)

Why have hair extensions?

Hair **extensions** are either natural human hair or man-made synthetic hair fibres. They can be applied either by using heated equipment to seal the extensions to hair (hot hair extension systems) or by using other methods to seal the extensions (cold hair extensions). Cold systems can be less damaging to the hair than hot systems. A client may consider asking for hair extensions for the following reasons.

- If their hair is thin or thinning.
- To increase the length of their hair.
- To add volume.
- To add different colours without committing.
- To add curls or straightness.

>> **Get up and go!**

You could try to interest clients in hair extensions by wearing them in your own hair. Try wearing some different textures, lengths and colours in your hair and take notice of the comments your clients make. Talk to them about the advantages of wearing extensions and show them some suitable styles.

Considering hair types when adding extensions

As you have learned, Caucasian/European and Asian/Oriental hair does differ due to the shape of the hair shaft, with Caucasian hair having an oval cross-section and Asian hair having a round cross-section. Hair can also be coarse, medium or fine. You will need to find out what type of hair your client has for the hair extension service to be successful.

You also need to be aware of the dangers of applying too much pressure on the hair when placing hair extensions. Hair that is excessively pulled can lead to a painful and irritable scalp, as well as hair breakage. If this pulling, or **tension**, continues the client may suffer from what is known as '**traction alopecia**', where the hair is pulled from the scalp due to excessive tension, leaving a bald area. This area will remain bald until new hair grows back through – it can be a month before you see only 1.25 cm of new hair.

Preparing the client for shampooing

You will need to comb through the client's hair to remove any tangles before shampooing. Use this time to check the client's scalp for cuts or irritated areas with the stylist. You will also need to discuss with the stylist the correct shampoo to use, which will probably be a clarifying shampoo that will remove all traces of product and leave the hair in its most natural state. Now might be a good time to advise the client not to shampoo their hair again for at least two days after the service. This is to give the hair **extensions** time to fully adhere to the hair shafts, allowing them to set properly.

Protecting the client and yourself

Protect the client's clothing with the appropriate towel, gown and waterproof cape. For your own protection, remember to wear personal protective equipment (PPE) when working with clients who are receiving a hair extension service. Your hands and clothing must be protected at all times. Wear the right type of gloves and apron when using hair extension removal products as they can burn through certain types of plastic.

Positioning the client and checking your own posture

As you prepare the client for the hair extension service, ask them whether or not they will need to move from the chair for any reason. The service may take several hours and so it is a good idea to find out if they have any physical needs you should be aware of. If they do need to get up and stretch or walk about during the service, you may like to offer them the opportunity to do so before you start any particularly tricky parts. Remember also to offer the client refreshments or a magazine before and regularly during the service.

As you will be working on the client for a long time, it is important to be aware of your own comfort. You should stand with straight legs and your feet slightly apart to maintain your balance. Keep your shoulders relaxed too. Taking these simple steps will help minimise your risk of developing injury and fatigue.

> **» Get up and go!**
>
> Think about the concerns usually experienced by clients when they have their hair extensions removed. What might they be worried about? How can you reassure them? Talk through your thoughts with your assessor.

> **» Get up and go!**
>
> Hair extension removal products 'melt' the bonds that hold the extensions in place, so they can also melt other plastics that they come into contact with. Think about the materials and tools you use on a daily basis in the salon that are made from plastic. How can they be protected from unnecessary damage? Discuss your thoughts with your assessor.

> **? Memory jogger**
>
> 1 Why might a client request hair extensions?
>
> 2 What causes traction alopecia?
>
> 3 Why must you make sure you are wearing the correct type of PPE when handling hair extension removal products?

Maintaining effective and safe methods of working when using hair extensions (2)

Keeping your work area clean and tidy

It is essential to keep your work area clean and tidy during the service. This will ensure the service runs smoothly and also presents a professional image to the client. Position tools and equipment for ease of use and prepare the trolley with all the resources you will need for removing hair **extensions**, ensuring they are clean and in good condition.

Working safely with hair extension products and tools

As with any product you use in the salon, always read the manufacturer's instructions and check with the stylist before using. Only make up the amount you need just before you need to use it. Some of the tools used when working with hair extensions, such as straighteners and the hot-bond hair extension system, often reach very high temperatures. Take great care when using these items to minimise the risk of accidents or injury.

Reducing the risk of cross-infection

Reduce the risk of cross-infection by being alert to any signs of infection and covering any open wounds or cuts with a suitable waterproof dressing. Report any personal infection or infestation to the appropriate member of staff. Always practise good standards of personal hygiene and wear clean, well-pressed clothes every day. Clients who have an open cut or wound must be treated with particular care. Seek advice from the stylist or your assessor and find out if barrier cream would be appropriate on this occasion. The situation may require your client to return for the service once the open wound has healed.

All tools and equipment used during the service must be cleaned in the appropriate way. Make sure you are familiar with how to clean or sterilise everything you have used, including brushes, combs, section clips, gowns and towels. You will also need to clean the applicator gun with the recommended cleaning product. This will reduce the risk of cross-infection and ensure tools and equipment are kept in good condition.

Reducing the risk of harm or injury to yourself, your colleagues and clients

Always keep a look out for hazards or risks which may arise during the course of the day. Clear away used product bottles and used materials such as bowls and cotton wool. Keep the floor clear from trailing cables, towels, gowns and cut hair, as well as items belonging to clients such as handbags, shopping bags, walking sticks and pushchairs. This will help to minimise the risk of any accidents occurring.

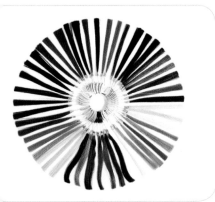

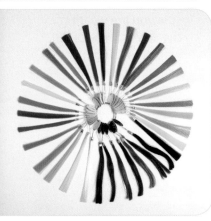

Hair extensions are available in different lengths and colours

Skin and suitability tests

A skin test should be carried out before the hair extension service is carried out. The gum-based products used in a cold hair extension system come into contact with the client's scalp, so sensitivity and allergy to these products must be tested. The test is carried out by applying a small amount of the product to the client's skin or by applying a hair extension using the product.

A suitability test allows the stylist to make sure the client's hair is suitable for the hair extension service. The stylist will also tell the client what is involved with looking after extensions and ask whether they can do this. Between three and five extensions may be placed in the hair, for an agreed fee, and then the client will return to the salon for a check-up, which will determine suitability in terms of:

- Is the hair strong enough to hold extensions for three months?
- Has there been any hair breakage?
- Are there any signs of scalp irritation?
- Does the client fully understand how to care for their extensions?

The results of any test must always be recorded on the client's record card.

Preparing the resources for applying or removing hair extensions

You will need to prepare a trolley for the stylist with the following items:

- client record card
- clean towels
- barrier cream
- gloves
- apron
- selection of combs
- old hairdressing scissors
- mixing mat[1]
- extension hair[1]
- bonding gun[1]
- resin sticks[1]
- heatproof drip mat[1]
- soft-bristled brush
- section clips
- removal tools[2]
- scalp protectors
- aftercare products and advice card/sheet
- cotton wool
- removal solutions
- hair dryer.

[1] For extension application
[2] For extension removal

All resources must be cleaned or sterilised after every use. This will help to minimise the risk of cross-infection.

>> **Get up and go!**

Find out how to prepare the hair extensions used in your salon by reading the manufacturer's instructions. Discuss the result, and how you found following the instructions, with a senior colleague.

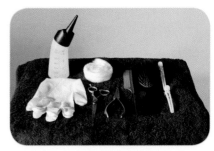

A trolley prepared for applying or removing hair extensions

? Memory jogger

1 Why is it important to work in a clean and tidy salon?
2 What does a suitability test involve and why is it carried out?
3 Name as many items as you can that are needed for a hair extension application service.

Removing hair extensions (1)

Before the appointment

When you have a client booked in to have their hair extensions removed, you will have to think about how long the extensions have been in the hair. It is recommended that hair extensions remain in place for no more than three months, but your client could be having them removed before or after this time. Hair grows about 1.25cm each month and the amount of growth since having the extensions applied can affect the removal service – extensions that have been in place for more than three months can be uncomfortable to remove. You might want to ask the client to apply conditioner to the bonds the night before their appointment, which will help break down the plastic resin, making the removal a little easier.

Preparing for the service

When your client is being prepared for the removal service, let them know it may feel like they are losing a lot of their hair as the extensions are removed. However, this hair loss will just be the hair they would have naturally shed over the time period they had the extensions. The client should also be made aware of how long the service will take. Depending on the type of hair extensions they have, it may take between 30 minutes and three hours.

You will need to prepare a trolley for the extension removal service. Items you will need in addition to those listed on page 193 are:

- **seal breakers**
- removal products
- cotton wool pads
- hairdryer
- seam releasers.

Make sure you wear suitable personal protective equipment throughout the service, to include gloves and an apron. Remember: hair extension removal products can be dangerous if you are not properly protected.

Items you will need in addition to those listed on page 193

>> **Get up and go!**

Why do you think a cotton wool pad is placed underneath the bond before applying the removal solution? Think about what the chemical does. Discuss your thoughts with your assessor.

Removing hair extensions as instructed by your stylist

First, you will need to separate the bonds one by one to make sure they have not become tangled together. You can then brush through the client's hair with a soft-bristled brush, working from the points of the hair through to the roots, being careful not to damage the natural hair. Take care not to apply too much tension while brushing through the roots as this may irritate the scalp.

The removal process for most extension systems will be similar to the ones described opposite but you should always check the manufacturer's instructions.

Removing hot hair extension systems

Section the client's hair and start the removal process on the hairline around the nape. Place a cotton wool pad underneath the hair extension bond and apply the removal solution, allowing it to penetrate the bond completely for the recommended time. This will soften the plastic bond, allowing the extension to be gently pulled away from the client's hair. Seal breakers may be needed before or after applying the removal solution, but this is dependent on the manufacturer's instructions.

Removing cold hair extension systems

Removing cold hair extensions follows a similar process to that described for hot hair extensions, except that the heat from a handheld hairdryer is used to activate the removal solution.

Check all hair extensions have been removed

Check each section as you work through your client's hair, making sure you have removed all of the hair extensions. Extensions can be quite small and easily missed when working amongst a mass of hair. When all the extensions have been removed, comb through each section gently, working from point to root. The stylist will need to check all the extensions have been removed, and when they are satisfied, your client is ready for the next part of the service.

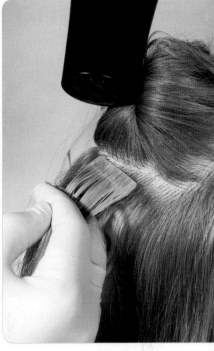

Using a hairdryer to speed up the removal of cold hair extensions

Best practice for removing hair extensions

- Always use products and equipment in line with the manufacturer's and stylist's instructions. Make sure you have understood any instructions given to you. If you are ever unsure, double-check.

- Always use tools and equipment for their intended purpose and make sure you know how to use them properly. You will then be able to use them effectively and minimise any damage to your client's hair.

- Keep in mind the client's comfort throughout the service. Regularly check their position and ask them if they need to move or stand up.

- Gel or conditioner can be used to protect the client's own hair when applying removal solution to the extensions.

- Make sure the removal solution doesn't run onto your client's face or clothes.

Removing hair extensions can be very uncomfortable or even painful for the client if it is not done correctly. The removal solution can irritate and damage skin and clothes so be especially careful when applying it. Take particular care around the eyes and consider using barrier cream around the hairline to prevent any solution running into the client's eyes. Always work in a well ventilated area as the removal solution can be very strong smelling. If you have any concerns at all during the service, always refer to your stylist for advice.

? Memory jogger

1 What is the recommended maximum time for wearing hair extensions?

2 Why might some of the client's hair come away with the hair extensions?

3 Why is a hairdryer used when removing some cold hair extensions?

4 Why is it important to check the client's hair for any stray hair extensions?

Removing hair extensions (2)

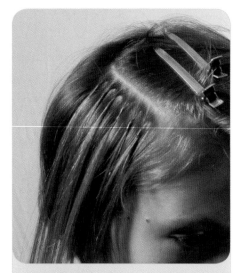

1 Prepare the trolley containing the tools and equipment needed for removing hair extensions

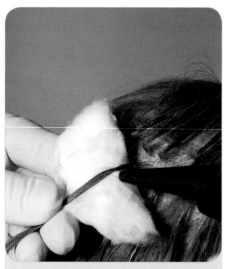

2 Wearing gloves to avoid any irritation, apply removal solution to soften the bond

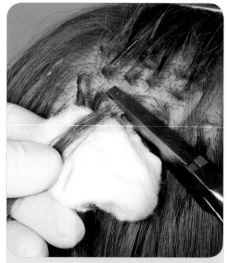

3 Break the bond with the seal breakers

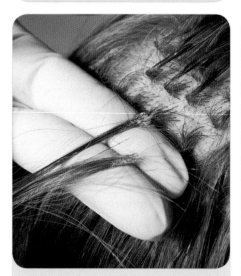

4 Pull the hair extension gently away from the scalp

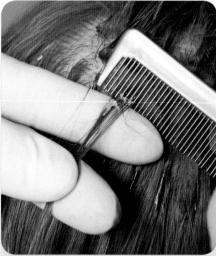

5 Use a fine tooth comb to remove excess softened glue

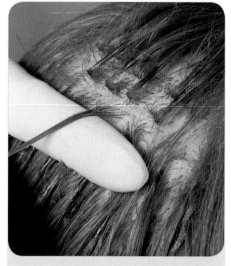

6 Continue to remove the remaining extensions

Shampooing the client's hair

The next part of the service, after the extensions have been removed, is a shampoo. This will remove all traces of the removal solution and bonding product, as well as any conditioner or gel you used to protect the client's hair. After shampooing, towel-dry the client's hair and scalp and make sure they are clean and free from products and excess moisture. Take the client to the styling area and comb through their hair, leaving it tangle-free without damaging the hair or scalp. Your client's hair is now ready for the next service, which may be more hair extensions!

Aftercare

You will need to advise your client how best to look after their new hair extensions at home. Tell them about any suitable products your salon sells and give them advice on appropriate hair care. The client should not rub their hair when shampooing and conditioning as this will cause the extensions to tangle with the client's own hair. Good aftercare advice will help the client maintain their extensions, make them want to return to your salon next time, and completes the hair extension service.

  Get up and go!

> Discuss with a colleague what a commercially acceptable timeframe is for removing hair extensions. Does this service appear on your salon price list?

Getting ready for assessment

Evidence requirements

You will be observed by your assessor on at least two occasions, one of which must include the removal of one hot and one cold extension system. You must also show that you have used two out of the four types of tools and products and removed both types of extensions from the range. This unit also includes an external paper.

What you must cover during your practical assessments

Ranges

1 Removal tools and products

2 Removal covers.

Performance criteria

In order to perform this unit successfully you must:

- maintain effective and safe methods of working when removing hair extensions
- remove hair extensions by following instructions from the stylist and minimising damage to the client's hair
- use specified tools and products effectively
- check your client's comfort at regular intervals throughout the service.

What you must know

In order to pass this unit, you will need to gather evidence to support a consistent performance with colleagues and clients. You should also collect evidence to show that you have taken part in self development activities over a period of time. This evidence will also be signed off in your candidate handbook, which you will be given by your assessor. This will be an official record to show that you have covered what you need to.

  Get ahead

Practise placing hair extensions on a male client. Applying a full head of hair extensions is time-consuming and requires neat and skilful work. You will need to think about a suitable colour, length, texture and style that are flattering to the client. Show your client some before and after photos and talk them through the process so they understand what will happen. Take some before and after photos of your client, as well as some photos of the process. You can use them to develop your portfolio, which can be used in your salon and at future interviews. You should aim to complete a full head of hair extensions on short to medium-length hair in less than four hours.

? Memory jogger

1 Why might you use gel or conditioner during the extension removal service?

2 Why shampoo the client's hair after removing extensions?

3 What aftercare advice could you give someone who has just had extensions applied?

Anatomy and physiology

In this section you will find the essential anatomy and physiology that you need to know to be able to carry out face and nail treatments for Level 1 Beauty Therapy.

As a beauty therapy assistant at Level 1 it is important to have a good knowledge of anatomy and physiology as many of the treatments that you will be learning about have an effect on the functioning and systems of the body. For example, massage of the face, hands and feet will improve the circulation, relax the muscles and improve the appearance of the skin.

In this unit you will learn about:

- Anatomy and physiology for facial treatments and make-up

- Anatomy and physiology for nail treatments.

Here are some key terms you may meet in this unit:

Sebum –
an oily substance secreted
from sebaceous glands

Physiology –
bodily processes

Impurities –
dirt and germs that can
cause bad health and
poor skin

Anatomy –
framework, structure of
the body, e.g. bones
and muscles

Functions –
purpose, job

Inflamed –
red and swollen, possibly
because of an infection

Elasticity –
stretchiness

Toxins –
poisons

Cranium –
the part of the skull that
encloses the brain

Secretes –
seeps, oozes

Nail bed –
the layer of cells on
which the nail plate rests

Nail grooves –
deep ridges that guide the
direction of nail growth

Lunula –
the half moon at the
base of the nail

Skull –
the part of the skeleton
that is found in the head

Nutrients –
vitamins and minerals

Anatomy and physiology for facial treatments and make-up [1]

Knowledge of **anatomy** and **physiology** for facial treatments and make-up will help you to understand the bone structure and shape of the face, because your make-up techniques and application methods should aim to enhance the face's natural shape. Facial treatments require massage of the face, neck and shoulder, so it is important to know about the muscles underneath the skin as well as the effect of ageing on the skin and how the skin **functions** keep it healthy.

The skin

The skin is a fascinating organ. Have a look at these facts about the largest organ of the body.

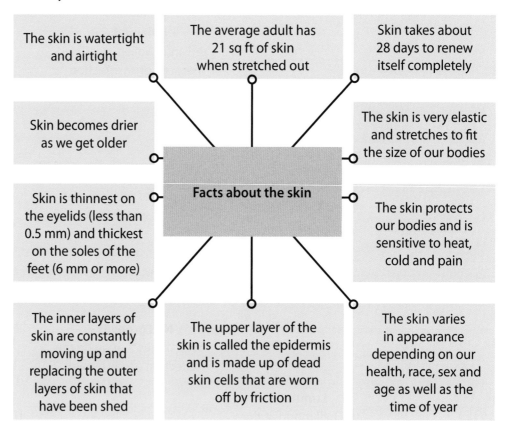

The skin is watertight and airtight

The average adult has 21 sq ft of skin when stretched out

Skin takes about 28 days to renew itself completely

Skin becomes drier as we get older

The skin is very elastic and stretches to fit the size of our bodies

Facts about the skin

Skin is thinnest on the eyelids (less than 0.5 mm) and thickest on the soles of the feet (6 mm or more)

The skin protects our bodies and is sensitive to heat, cold and pain

The inner layers of skin are constantly moving up and replacing the outer layers of skin that have been shed

The upper layer of the skin is called the epidermis and is made up of dead skin cells that are worn off by friction

The skin varies in appearance depending on our health, race, sex and age as well as the time of year

Amazing facts about the skin

The structure of the skin

The skin has three main layers:

- the epidermis
- the dermis
- the fatty layer.

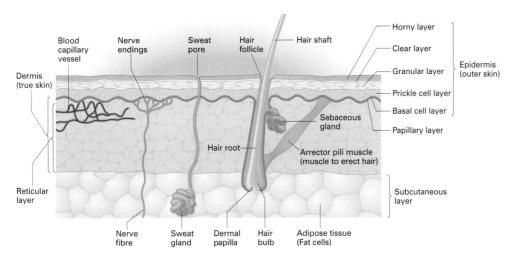

The structure of the skin

The upper layer of the skin (epidermis) is made up of five layers. Each layer has a different job to do in order to keep the skin healthy. It is not essential that you know about the five layers of skin at Level 1, but it may be useful to understand a little about them.

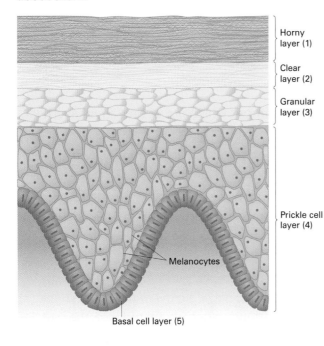

Look at the table below. You may find it easier to remember and say the English names rather than the Latin ones. It may also be helpful to know that *stratum* is the Latin word for layer.

The five layers of the epidermis

The five layers of the epidermis are as follows.

Layer	Latin name	English name
Layer 1	Stratum corneum	Horny layer
Layer 2	Stratum lucidum	Clear layer
Layer 3	Stratum granulosum	Granular layer
Layer 4	Stratum spinosum	Prickle cell layer
Layer 5	Stratum germinativum	Basal cell layer

Anatomy and physiology for facial treatments and make-up (2)

The skin

Knowing about the structure of the skin can help us to understand its **functions**.

> **» Get up and go!**
>
> Make a card game or board game that will help you to remember the parts of the skin, the functions of the skin or some facts about skin. Be adventurous and creative.
>
> Once you have created your game, play it with other students in your class. A card game could be based around the structure of the skin, with each card having the correct name of the skin layer on one side and on the other the function it has. It is up to you how you design your game, but the most important thing is that it helps you to remember things based around anatomy and physiology.

Functions of the skin

The skin does many important jobs, without which our bodies could overheat, become ill and get injured easily.

- Vitamin production – the sun's rays on the skin make vitamin D for the body. This vitamin is needed for strong bones and teeth.

- Sense and feeling – the nerve endings in our skin are very sensitive. They pick up changes in temperature or pressure, and alert us to pain. Messages are quickly sent from the nerve endings to our brain so that we can respond – for example, by stopping the source of the pain.

- Heat control – skin helps to control the temperature in our body, e.g. how hot or cold we are. When we are too hot, we begin to sweat through sweat glands in our skin, and this cools us down. When we are too cold, the muscles that are joined to the hairs in our skin cause goose pimples and we begin to shiver, which warms up the body. The correct temperature of the skin should be about 36°C.

- Absorption – the skin is able to absorb small amounts of products that are put on the skin.

- Protection – skin is like a waterproof jacket as it provides the body with protection from dirt, bacteria and injury. To keep the outer layers of skin smooth and soft and free from splits and cracks that would let germs enter, the body produces oil through the skin's pores.

- Excretion – some waste products and **toxins** are removed from the body through our sweat.
- Secretion – the skin **secretes** a substance through its pores called **sebum**, which keeps our skin smooth and supple.
- Storage – the skin stores fat and water, without which we could not survive.

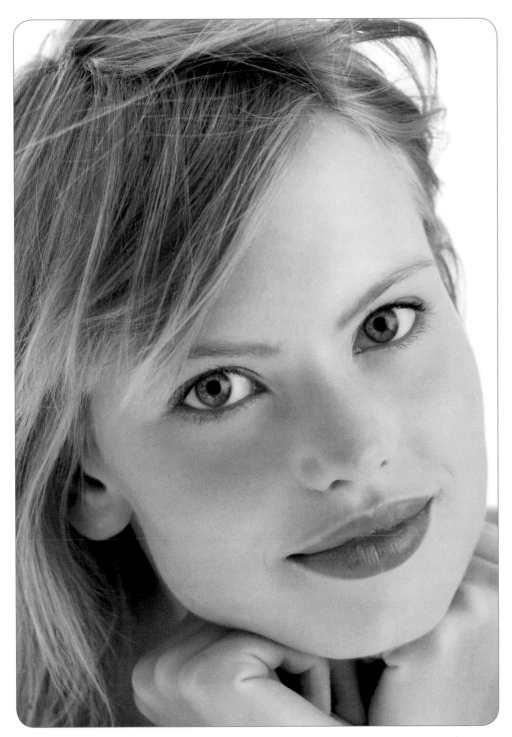

The skin does many important jobs, so make sure you look after yours

? Memory jogger

1 How many layers of the epidermis are there?

A 3

B 4

C 5

D 6

2 What are the functions of the skin?

Anatomy and physiology for facial treatments and make-up (3)

The skin

Healthy skin

Given all of the jobs that our skin does, it is easy to understand why it is so important to look after it. The skin on our faces can reveal how healthy we are. When we are healthy our skin glows, and when we are ill the effects can be seen in the colour and condition of our faces. The skin can also reflect how we feel – when we are fed up, stressed or have an illness, the skin becomes dull and lifeless. As we get older, facial skin can reveal the sort of life we have lived.

If we have sunbathed too much	the skin will be thickened, orangey yellow and very lined
If we have smoked	the skin around the mouth will have lines from sucking on the cigarette, and the nose and cheeks may be red with broken veins from the heat and smoke of the cigarette
If we have cried or laughed a lot	the fine skin around the eyes can be very wrinkled
If we have frowned a lot	we may have deep ridges in between our eyebrows
When we are dehydrated	our skin becomes dry and flaky
When we have a temperature	the skin flushes and becomes sweaty
When we feel sick	the skin looks pale and grey
If we eat an unhealthy diet	we may have blotchy, spotty skin

How our actions affect our skin

The skin varies in appearance depending on our sex, age and race as well as changing in different seasons. Our diet, health and lifestyle also affect our skin so it is important to remember to care for it and treat it well throughout our life. Skin that is cared for well in teenage years will mean healthier and more attractive skin when you are in your 50s and 60s.

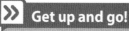
Get up and go!

Think about members of your family, both male and female, old and young. What do you notice about their skin? Write down your observations and then discuss them in groups.

Tips for healthy skin

Here are some tips for healthy skin. You may want to mention some of these in the aftercare advice you give to your clients.

Weather

Protect the skin with creams that contain a UV-filter (at least SPF 15) when in the sun and use a rich moisturiser in cold weather.

Exercise

Exercise improves the body's circulation (the blood flow around the body) which in turn improves the skin's colour and texture.

Alcohol and drugs

These cause dehydration, which dries out the skin. They also result in the body losing important **nutrients** that the skin needs to work properly.

Smoking

Smoking ages and dries out the skin, and causes tiny broken blood vessels to appear. If you don't smoke, stay away from smoky areas.

Cleansing

It is important to keep the skin clean by cleansing every day. This prevents germs from building up and causing an infection. In addition, a dirty complexion is unattractive and looks unhealthy.

Sleep

It is important that you get plenty of sleep, because when you sleep your skin rests and repairs itself.

What you eat

It is important to eat a balanced diet that includes lots of fresh fruit and vegetables, and all of the vitamins and minerals that your body needs.

Water

Drink lots of water daily – about eight glasses. Water flushes out **impurities** from the body, which helps to keep the skin clear and prevents it from drying out.

Ageing

As the skin gets older it loses moisture and **elasticity**, so it is important to take care of the skin from a young age by using moisturisers and gentle skin care.

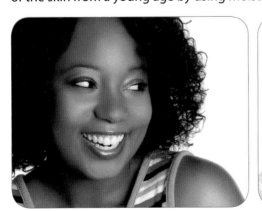

Young skin   Mature skin

? Memory jogger

1 How does exercise improve the skin's colour and texture?

2 As the skin ages, it loses:
   A Elasticity
   B Cleanliness
   C Colour
   D Impurities

3 When does your skin rest and repair itself?
   A During the daytime
   B During exercise
   C After mealtimes
   D During sleep

4 How does dehydration affect the skin?
   A It makes it oily
   B It makes it shiny
   C It makes it flaky
   D It makes it dirty

Anatomy and physiology for facial treatments and make-up [4]

Muscles and bones of the face and head

Underneath the skin are muscles and bones.

- The muscles allow for facial movement, and each facial muscle produces a different movement.
- The bones provide support for the muscles, and protect the brain and facial organs from injury.

The muscles and bones also give shape to the face. When carrying out make-up treatments your techniques should aim to enhance the natural shape.

Muscles

Many of the muscles found on the face are very small and attached to other muscles. For Level 1 you do not need to know the correct names and actions of the muscles, but the diagram below will help you to understand the face better when you carry out practical treatments.

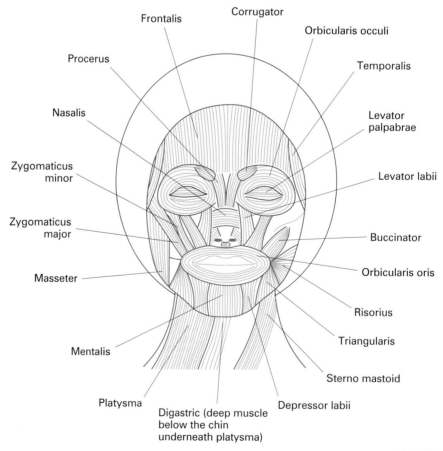

Muscles of the face and neck

When we make different facial expressions such as smiling, laughing or frowning, the muscles pull our faces into different shapes, as shown in the diagram below.

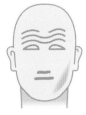

1. FRONTALIS
Amazement, wonder, shock

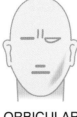

2. ORBICULARIS OCULI
Deep thought

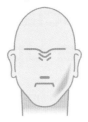

3. PROCERUS
Threatening, unfriendliness, anger

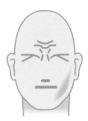

4. CORRUGATOR
Sadness and sorrow, regret

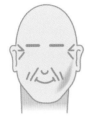

5. ZYGOMATICUS MAJOR
Laughter

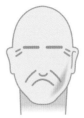

6. LEVATOR LABII SUPERIORIS
Grief, discontented

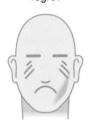

7. LEVATOR LABII
Extreme grief with tears

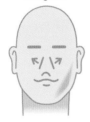

8. COMPRESSOR NARIS
Concentration, interest and attention or anger and violent behaviour

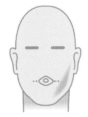

9. ORBICULARIS ORIS
Pouting, smoking, kissing

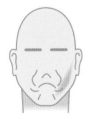

10. DEPRESSOR ANGULIORIS
Dislike, disapproval

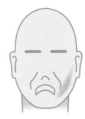

11. DEPRESSOR LABII INFERIORIS
Disgust

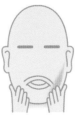

12. PLATYSMA
Anger, pain, torture or hard work

The actions of different facial muscles in facial expressions

 Get ahead

Copy the 12 facial expressions in the diagram above. See if you can work out which muscles are being used for each expression. It will help if you make faces at each other.

》 Get up and go!

Mould some plasticine into the shape of facial muscles using this book to guide you. Place it over a model of a skeleton.

Anatomy and physiology for facial treatments and make-up (5)

The bones of the head, otherwise known as the **skull**, keep the muscles in place and protect the brain and other parts of the head from injury. The skull is made up of the **cranium** and the lower jaw (mandible). There are 22 bones in the skull in total. Eight of these make up the cranium, as shown in the table below.

Bone	Position
1 x ethmoid bone	At the roof of the nose
1 x frontal bone	Forms the front of the cranium, forehead and upper eye sockets
1 x occipital bone	At the back and lower part of the cranium
2 x parietal bones	At the back and top of the cranium
1 x sphenoid bone	At the base of the cranium, in front of the temporal bones
2 x temporal bones	At the side, around the ears

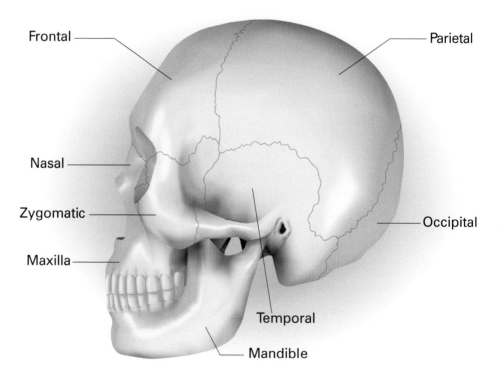

The bones of the skull

The face

The bones of the face also protect the soft tissues inside the head. The face is made up of 14 bones. The seven main ones are shown in the table below.

Bone	Position
1 x mandible	This is the lower jaw and is the only moving bone in the face. It enables movement of the mouth for chewing and talking
2 x maxillae	These form the upper jaw, most of the side wall of the nose and the front part of the soft palate (the top of the mouth)
2 x nasal bones	These form the bridge (upper part) of the nose
2 x zygomatic bones	These form the cheekbones

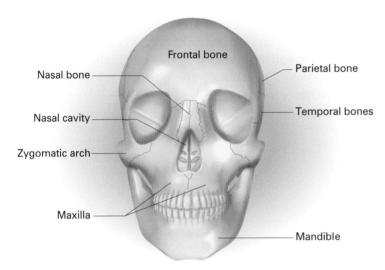

The bones of the face

How the bones affect facial shape

The photo below shows a person with prominent (noticeable) cheekbones. The bones that create this are called the zygomatic bones and some people have less prominent ones than others. The line of the chin and jaw is decided by the mandible bone. The shape of the nose is decided by the nasal bones. All of the bones in our face and head shape us.

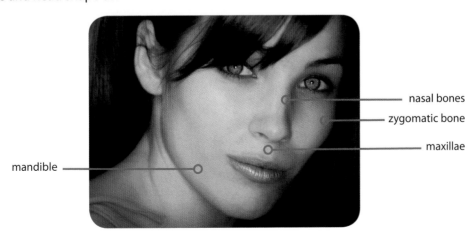

The bones of the face affect its shape

? Memory jogger

1 How many bones are there in the face?

   A 5

   B 8

   C 14

   D 22

2 Which bone forms the forehead?

3 Which bone might you apply cheek colour to?

   A Maxilla

   B Mandible

   C Zygomatic

   D Occipital

4 Name one function of bone.

Anatomy and physiology for nail treatments (1)

In the same way that knowing about the bones and structure of the face is helpful for facial treatments, understanding the structure of the hand and nails is useful knowledge for nail treatments. The structure of the nail and how to keep it healthy is valuable information to pass on to clients, whereas knowledge of the muscles and structure of the hand is useful for massage therapies.

The nails

The structure of nails

The nails grow from the ends of the fingers and toes. The nail plate is a hard, rectangular and curved structure made up of flat layers of cells. It covers and protects the sensitive fingertips and **nail bed**. When healthy a nail should be pink, smooth and flexible with a white free edge that shows no signs of flaking or splitting. The cuticle should not be dry, rough or **inflamed**.

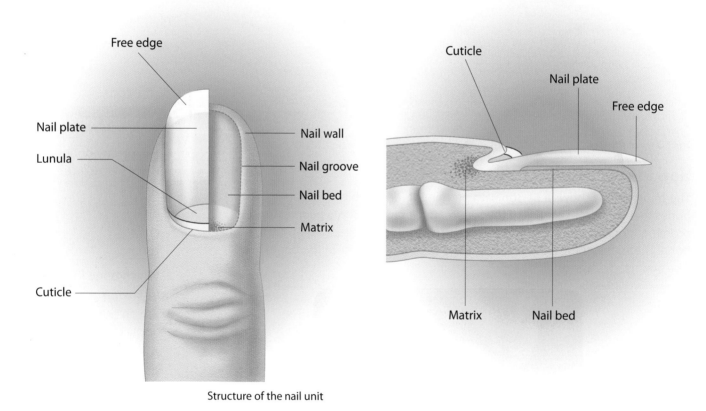

Structure of the nail unit

Parts and functions of the nail

Matrix

The matrix is the only living part of the nail. Its function is to grow and replace the cells that form the nail. The quality, strength and health of the nail is therefore decided in the matrix. The nail's condition depends on how healthy the cell growth is and whether or not there has been any damage to the matrix, such as from knocks, injury (for example, a nail being shut in the door), poor treatment or an infection. However, as long as the matrix has not been permanently damaged, the effect on the nail is usually only temporary.

Lunula

The **lunula** is also known as the half moon. It is found on all nails, but on some it is easier to see. It is at the base of the nails and is the visible part of the matrix.

Nail bed

The **nail bed** is the healthy soft tissue underneath the nail plate. It gives the nail its pink appearance. It contains blood vessels and nerve endings. Ridges in the nail bed help to keep the nail firmly in place as it grows.

Nail plate

The nail plate lies on top of the nail bed and is the main part of the nail. It is pink in colour because of the soft tissue underneath, which is visible through the plate. The nail plate is made up of layers of fat, moisture and growth cells, and these give the nail its strength. If you tear part of the nail off, it is very painful because it is attached to blood vessels and nerve endings.

Free edge

The free edge is the hardest part of the nail. It grows past the end of the nail bed and fingertip. It is whitish in colour, as it has grown beyond the pink tissue. If you break this part of the nail, it does not hurt because it is not joined to blood vessels or nerve endings.

Nail grooves or nail wall

The **nail grooves** are deep ridges that lie along the back and sides of the nail. The grooves at the side of the nail guide the direction of the nail growth. The grooves also help to stop germs from entering the nail bed. If the nail grooves are not kept soft and well-moisturised, hangnails can appear.

These are dry strips of skin at the sides of the nail that can become very sore and **inflamed** if left untreated or pulled off.

Cuticle

The cuticle is found at the base of the nail. It is designed to protect the matrix against germs by forming a barrier. You should never cut the cuticle off during a manicure, as the matrix could become infected.

Anatomy and physiology for nail treatments [2]

The nails

Nail health

The state of your nails can provide the secret to your health. A doctor can often tell what illness a person has by looking at the appearance of the nails. For example, some nail conditions can show that a person has heart problems, poor circulation or a lack of iron.

Nail facts

1   The nails are held together with fats and moisture. You can peel back one or two layers when the nails are out of condition.

2   Nails dry out as we get older.

3   The ridges on a nail are natural and are there to help the nail plate stick to the **nail bed**. If the nails are filed or buffed to get a smooth look, this will weaken the nail. However, very deep ridges can be a sign of illness.

4   Fingernails take 3 to 6 months to grow from root to tip.

5   Toenails take 10 to 12 months to grow from root to tip.

6   On average, nails grow one eighth of an inch (0.3 cm) per month.

7   Nails grow faster in the summer than in the winter.

8   If a person is right-handed, his or her fingernails will grow faster on the right hand than on the left hand. This is because the person's right hand gets more stimulation. (The reverse is true for left-handed people.)

9   Men's nails grow faster than women's nails.

10 The longer the finger, the faster the nail growth.

11 Of the nails on the hand, the smallest fingernail grows the slowest, and the thumb nail grows the second slowest.

12 Nails grow faster in younger people.

13 If we restrict our diet too much, our nail growth slows down.

14 If left to grow too long, the nails start to curl.

>> **Get up and go!**

Describe how you think your hands and nails should look when giving a treatment, so that a client will not be put off but will feel confident that she is being treated by a person who knows what she is doing.

Bones of the hand and wrist

There are three sections to the bones of the hand and wrist. These are:

- the carpals in the wrist, consisting of eight bones
- the metacarpals in the hand or palm – there is one metacarpal on each finger and thumb
- the phalanges in the fingers and thumbs – there are three phalanges that make up each finger and two phalanges on the thumb.

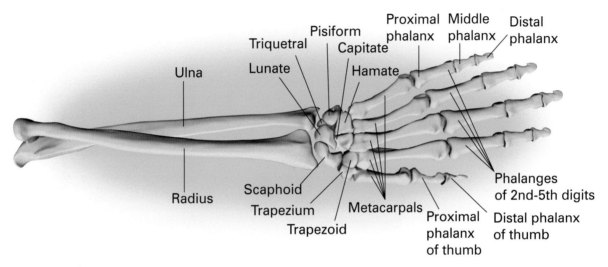

The bones of the hand and wrist

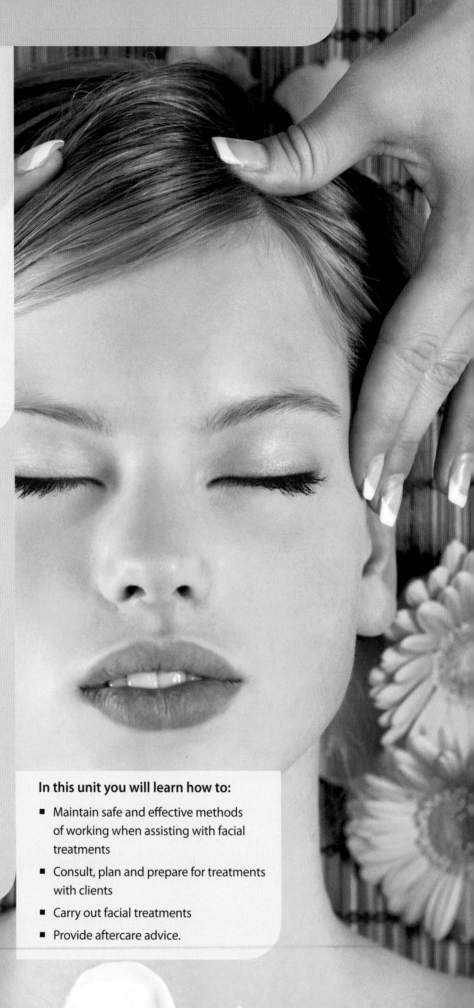

UNIT B2

Assist with facial skin care treatments

Facial skin goes through many changes over the years. Our faces are under constant pressure from the weather and dirt in the environment, and also undergo a natural ageing process. Only some of us are lucky enough to have a naturally clear complexion that will not become too lined as we get older. We can cover up other parts of our body if they are less than perfect, but this is not so with our faces. Our faces are on show all the time and it is therefore important that we look after them. Nothing beats regular facials when it comes to keeping our skin glowing and healthy. Facial treatments are essential for thorough cleansing of the skin and increased cell renewal.

In this unit you will learn how to assist with facial skin care treatments. You will also learn how to prepare for treatments and about ways to improve the skin through the correct use of skin care products. At all times during facial skin care treatments you will also need to follow effective health, safety and hygiene procedures.

In this unit you will learn how to:

- Maintain safe and effective methods of working when assisting with facial treatments
- Consult, plan and prepare for treatments with clients
- Carry out facial treatments
- Provide aftercare advice.

Here are some key terms you may meet in this unit:

Complexion –
skin tone, texture and colour

Contra-actions –
unwanted reactions
to a treatment

Pores –
tiny openings in the skin
that produce oil to
moisturise the skin

Effleurage –
to flow, so these are
stroking, smooth
massage movements

Comedone extractor –
a tool for blackhead removal

Petrissage –
to knead, so these are
circling, kneading
massage movements

Rehydrate –
add water or moisture

Moisturise –
soften and rehydrate by
the use of creams

Eczema –
a dry skin condition
that shows up as
rough, flaky skin

Tapotement –
a stimulating form of massage
using cupping or pinching
movements

Astringent –
strong solution to
cleanse the skin

Contra-indications –
conditions that make the
client unsuitable for treatment
such as skin infections or high
blood pressure

Dehydration –
lacking in water

Allergies –
reactions, sensitivity

Client consultation –
question-and-answer sessions
with a client that are designed
to find out information
about them

Blemishes –
skin marks

Conjunctivitis –
an eye infection

Maintain safe and effective methods of working when assisting with facial treatments [1]

As with all beauty therapies, skin care treatments involve close work with the client and require close attention from you. Safe working practices are very important and you must make sure you follow much higher standards of hygiene than you might ever think of doing at home. You should also know that some facial treatments use electrical equipment, and therefore when you are assisting a therapist you need to be able to recognise safe working methods and follow instructions from the therapist.

The work area

Many different products, tools and pieces of equipment are needed for a facial treatment and you will need to set up your work area with these items before you bring your client to the treatment room. These items are listed and explained on pages 220–223.

The most important thing to remember is that when carrying out or assisting with a facial treatment, you need to be both safe and effective. This means that your work area must always be:

- organised – nothing forgotten, all equipment and tools on a trolley, set up in the order of when it will be used
- easy to reach – you will not have to overstretch to reach it or walk across the room
- hygienic – everything cleaned, disinfected and sterilised, and your couch or chair has a protective cover.

Good organisation with careful consideration of your client's needs is the key to successful preparation and a well thought out workspace for skin care treatments.

> **» Get up and go!**
>
> Take two or three photographs of work area set-ups using your mobile phone or digital camera. Upload them to a computer and see how many mistakes there are and which is the best prepared work area. Discuss your findings with your group. You could also insert the photos in a PowerPoint presentation so it is easy for the whole group to look at and make comments on.

Sterilisation and cleaning of skin care tools and equipment

As for any salon treatment, you need to maintain accepted industry hygiene practices throughout a facial treatment. Following the correct hygiene methods will prevent cross-infection, which is when germs or bacteria are transferred from one person to other, sometimes with nasty results such as skin and eye infections.

Unit G20 explains in detail how germs and bacteria can be passed on during treatments and what you should do to prevent this from happening, so refer back to pages 26–27. The table below shows how cross-infection could occur during a facial treatment and will help you to understand what hygiene means in practical terms for this particular treatment.

Stage of the facial treatment	Unhygienic practices that could lead to cross-infection
Preparing to treat the client and/or during the whole of the treatment	Completing a treatment on one client and then carrying straight on to the next client without washing your hands, or going to the toilet during the treatment and returning to the client without washing your hands
Removing blackheads	Not sterilising the blackhead extractor
Applying a mask	Not washing and sterilising the mask brush
Applying moisturiser	Using your fingers instead of a disposable spatula to scoop out the cream from the pot, meaning that after a few treatments the cream is full of germs from different clients

Facial treatments use quite a lot of disposable products such as cotton wool, tissues, spatulas, mask sponges, orange sticks and couch roll. Non-disposable items need to be prepared carefully for use.

- Equipment such as steamers, trolleys and magnifying lamps should be wiped over with disinfectant before and after use and metal tools such as blackhead extractors need to be sterilised.

- Mask brushes should be washed in warm soapy water, left to air dry and then placed in an ultraviolet cabinet.

- All skincare products should be removed from their containers using a spatula or orange stick.

 Top tip

Do not scoop out creams with your fingers, as this contaminates the whole pot. Always use a clean spatula.

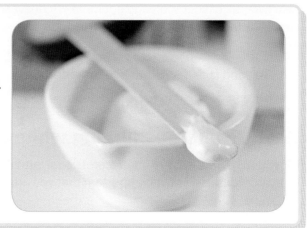

Maintain safe and effective methods of working when assisting with facial treatments (2)

Maintaining hygiene throughout

Hygiene is not something that you only need to think about before beginning a treatment. Throughout any treatment, you must ensure that you maintain the same high standards. This applies to the tools, equipment and products that you use, and also to your own personal hygiene. Remember the following rules.

- If you sneeze or cough you must cover your mouth and turn away from the client and then go and wash your hands.
- If you blow your nose, wash your hands.
- Don't put fingers in pots and containers.
- Keep your work area tidy.
- Throw away used tissues and cotton wool immediately in a nearby foot pedal bin.

>> Get up and go!

Make a checklist of how your skin and make-up should look so that a client will not be put off, but will instead feel confident that she is being treated by a person who knows what she is doing.

Leaving the work area clean and tidy

Remember that a tidy and clean work area is not only important for health and safety, it also shows that the salon is professional and run properly. A dirty, untidy room is an instant turn-off for any client because it demonstrates a lack of care and hygiene. After you have finished the treatment and your client has left, you must clear away all of your tools and equipment to leave your work area clean and tidy and ready for the next client. This will include:

- wiping over trolleys, couches, bins and stools with disinfectant
- washing facial tools and equipment
- putting bedding in to be laundered.

Posture and positioning while working

For you to be able to carry out a professional treatment and for the treatment to be enjoyable for the client, it is important that you are both comfortable.

A facial treatment is typically carried out while the client lies on a comfortable couch. The client may lie completely flat or semi-inclined and must be positioned comfortably. Your client should be able to remain relaxed during the treatment without having to twist or move so that you can reach her.

For you, bad posture will cause physical aches and pains. In addition, the treatment will probably not be as good because it has been carried out in an awkward position.

You will need to decide whether you will stand or sit behind the couch. It depends on:

- the height and angle of the couch – whether it is flat or sloping
- your height and whether you can reach the client if you sit down.

Adjust the height of the couch so that you don't have to reach too far up or down, and make sure that all the equipment and tools you need are within easy reach. It is very important that you do not overstretch your neck and back to reach tools or the client's face because you will end up with a long-term back problem. Overstretching will also affect the muscles and veins in your legs and could possibly cause varicose veins over time.

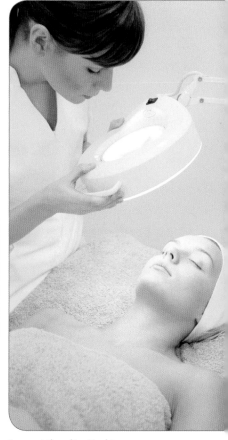

Inspect the client's skin under a bright light

 Top tip

When standing for long periods of time, move a little to keep the circulation going. For example, every now and then:

- move from one foot to the other
- bend the knee back a few times, then repeat on the other foot.

Environmental conditions

Lighting

Lighting must be bright and clear for the skin inspection, but soft and relaxing for the rest of the facial treatment. A light that can be dimmed is ideal, along with a magnifying lamp for inspection work.

Ambience

This means the atmosphere or mood that is created within the treatment room or salon. This is important because the aim is to get the client to relax and enjoy her treatment and the whole experience.

Relaxing music, pleasant-smelling oils and scented candles can all act to create a favourable atmosphere.

Heating and ventilation

The facial treatment area needs to be warm and inviting. It is usual during a facial for a client to become cold. This is because when they relax their body temperature can drop. For this reason it is necessary to have covers that can be placed on the client, such as a blanket or duvet, as well as keeping the temperature of the room fairly warm. Thermostatically controlled central heating is the best, as heaters that you need to turn on and off when needed are not very efficient.

? Memory jogger

1 What sort of lighting is needed to carry out facial treatments?

2 Why is posture important when carrying out a treatment?

3 How can relaxing affect a client's temperature?

4 What is the best form of heating in a treatment room?

Consult, plan and prepare for treatments with clients [1]

Before beginning any skin care treatment, you need to make sure that both you and the client are well prepared. You will need to chat to your client about why she would like a facial, record the client's contact details and information about her skin and her home skin care routine, and carry out a simple analysis to help you to decide the skin type, identify any problems and be able to plan a treatment suitable for the client.

However, the first step before collecting your client and bringing her to the treatment room is to set up your work area with all the materials that you will need. These are:

- basics – the disposable products, laundry and workspace requirements
- tech tools – the tools, such as tweezers and scissors, that you will need
- products – all the creams and lotions needed for the treatment.

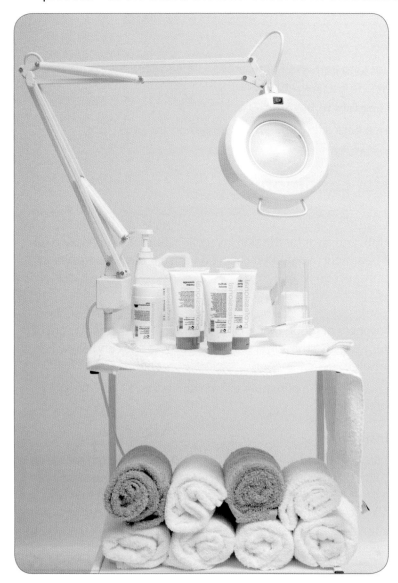

What you need to carry out a facial skin care treatment

Basics

When setting up for a facial skin care treatment, make sure you have all the basics to hand.

Item	Purpose
Dampened cotton wool	Cotton wool squares: for removing cleanser and putting on toner. They need to be large enough to wrap around your first two fingers.
	Cotton wool half moons: these are placed under the bottom eyelashes, to protect the skin under the eyes from the make-up that is being cleaned off.
	Eye pads (circles or squares): these rest on the eye while using the magnifying lamp for skin inspection or blackhead removal. They can be soaked in witch hazel to soothe the eyes while the client is wearing a face mask.
Dry cotton wool	To cover the tip of an orange stick for removing eye make-up.
Split tissues	To blot excess toner or moisturiser. Tissues are normally two-ply – this means that each tissue is made up of two very thin layers. For the purpose of beauty treatments, however, tissues are split as this makes them more economical to use and easier to curve around the shape of the face.
Sponges	These can be used with warm water to remove mask products from the skin. However, they are not easy to clean and sterilise. They need to be washed in very hot soapy water, dried thoroughly and then placed in an ultraviolet sterilising cabinet. The other option is for a salon to charge enough for a facial so that the sponge can be given to the client at the end of her treatment. Otherwise, it is best to use damp cotton wool squares for mask removal.
Towels	You will need one hand towel to dry your own hands during the treatment, one medium-sized towel for placing across the client's chest, and one large towel for covering her body during the treatment (if a blanket is not used).
Blanket	In the winter months, a honeycomb blanket may be needed to keep the client warm during the treatment.
Fitted couch sheet	To protect the couch from marks and product spills during a treatment.
Couch roll	This is used to cover the fitted couch sheet so that it does not need to be washed after each treatment. It is also used to protect the towel lying over the client's chest, and the pillow and the headband from skin care and mask products.
Headband or turban	This is used to protect the client's hair from the products and to prevent her hair from getting in the way of the treatment.
Gown	As the client needs to remove her top clothing, you may need to give her a gown to wear to prevent any embarrassment.
Waste bin	A pedal bin with a lid is best for hygiene purposes, as you can open it without touching it with your hands.
Sterilising jar	This should be filled with antiseptic or disinfectant solution, so that small metal tools such as blackhead extractors and tweezers can be placed in it during the treatment. The solution will help to keep germ levels down, but it will not destroy germs completely. The solution should be changed after every client.
Dishes	Small plastic or metal dishes are needed to hold cotton wool and tissues, as well as the client's jewellery.

 Top tips

How to prepare dampened cotton wool squares:

- Cut squares approximately 80 cm² in size from a cotton wool roll.
- Take about four to six squares and hold them between the palms of your hands under a running tap. When they are soaked through, squeeze out the water so that they are only damp and not dripping.
- Peel back thin layers from your thick pad of cotton wool. You should have about 16–20 pads. These are your facial pads for removing and applying products.

 Top tip

Each salon has its own way of preparing a client for a treatment, so you will need to find out how your workplace sets up, for example, whether they use sheets and blankets, or towels.

Consult, plan and prepare for treatments with clients (2)

Potions

When setting up for a facial skin care treatment, you need to make sure that you have different types of products to suit different skin types. You will learn how to determine a client's skin type on page 228.

Product	Purpose	Types
Eye make-up remover	These are mild cleansing products that dissolve eye make-up so that it can be easily wiped off without rubbing the eyes.	Eye make-up remover is available as an oil, lotion or gel. Some remove waterproof make-up.
Cleansers	To remove old make-up. To clean dirt, dust and grime from the skin and **pores**. To remove oil and dead skin cells.	Cream – this thick, creamy cleanser is used for dry or mature skin types. It dissolves make-up quickly. Milk – this is a thin, runny cleanser that can be used on most skin types except very dry skin. It is ideal for young or normal skin types, but is not very good at removing heavy or waterproof make-up. Lotion – this is similar in thickness to a milk cleanser but includes ingredients to help spotty and combination skins, which are usually found in younger clients. Facial washes – these can be liquids, gels or lotions. They are gently rubbed into the skin with some water to make a lather. Facial washes can be used on any skin as long as moisturiser is applied afterwards, as the skin can feel quite tight. Facial washes are especially good for men and people who like to feel freshly washed.
Toners	To remove any left-over cleanser from the skin. To dissolve oil. To refresh and cool the skin. To tighten the skin and pores.	Toners come in different strengths and are chosen depending on the skin type. The main ingredients are water, alcohol, colour and perfume. The greater the alcohol content, the stronger the toner. Toners for oily problem skins are called **astringents** and have the highest alcohol content.
Face masks*	Face masks are usually applied towards the end of a facial, after the skin has been cleansed, steamed and massaged. A mask should never be applied to skin that has not been thoroughly cleansed. Depending on the ingredients, face masks can: • deep clean the skin and pores • remove oil and dead skin cells • deeply **moisturise** and nourish the skin • tighten the pores • soften fine lines • soothe sensitive skins.	Setting – these masks are usually made of clay powder. They are mixed with distilled water or toner to make a paste that can be painted on the skin with a mask brush. Non-setting – these masks can be creams or gels in a tube or pot. Specialised – these are nourishing warm oil masks or deeply moisturising paraffin wax masks. Food – just as the name says, these face masks can be made using ingredients from your own fridge at home.
Moisturisers	To soften and protect the skin's surface. To **rehydrate** the skin. To help the application of make-up by providing a smooth base.	As with cleansers, moisturisers can be: • creams for dry skins • lotions for oily skins • milks for young, normal or sensitive skins.

* For Level 1 you only need to know how to use a ready-made non-setting face mask. However, it is helpful if you have a basic knowledge of the other types that you might see being used in the salon.

» Get up and go!

Try out these recipes for food masks.

For dry skin

Mash avocado, add egg yolk and mix until creamy. Apply to the face with a spatula. Leave for 10–15 minutes, then rinse off.

For oily skin

Mix oatmeal and honey together, then apply to the face with a spatula. Leave for 10–15 minutes, then rinse off.

When using food ingredients, you should use the masks as soon as you have made them, as they can go off very quickly. Only use eggs with the Lion mark.

Tech tools

When setting up for a facial skin care treatment, you need to prepare all the tools you will need.

Item	Purpose
Spatula	A spatula is a wide wooden stick that is used to scoop out cream or lotion from pots. Fingers should never be used, as this is very unhygienic and could result in cross-infection. A spatula is also used to tuck the client's hair into a headband instead of your fingers.
Orange sticks	These are made of orange wood, which is slightly bendy. One end is pointed and the other end is shaped like a hoof. Both ends of the orange stick are coated in cotton wool for hygiene purposes, as the cotton wool can be removed and thrown away after use. The cotton wool softens the tip for safety when cleaning around the eyes.
Comedone extractor	This loop-end tool is designed to remove blackheads. It is pressed onto a blackhead, then steady, gentle pressure is applied. If the blackhead is ready, its contents will pop out.
Mask brush	This is usually a strong bristle brush that is used to paint the mask on to the skin. Some brushes are fan shaped. They are very hard to sterilise completely, so care must be taken to wash them thoroughly with hot soapy water, leave them to dry and then place them in an ultraviolet sterilising cabinet for the recommended time. Alternatively, a disposable spatula can be used to apply some masks.

? Memory jogger

1 Moisturisers are used to:

   A Hydrate the skin

   B Tone the skin

   C Wash the skin

   D Exfoliate the skin

2 Give three types of face masks that can be used.

3 The best type of cleanser for oily to combination skins is:

   A Milk

   B Lotion

   C Cream

   D Facial wash

4 How does eye make-up remover work to remove eye make-up?

5 List three tech tools that you will need to set up for a facial.

Consult, plan and prepare for treatments with clients (3)

Client consultation

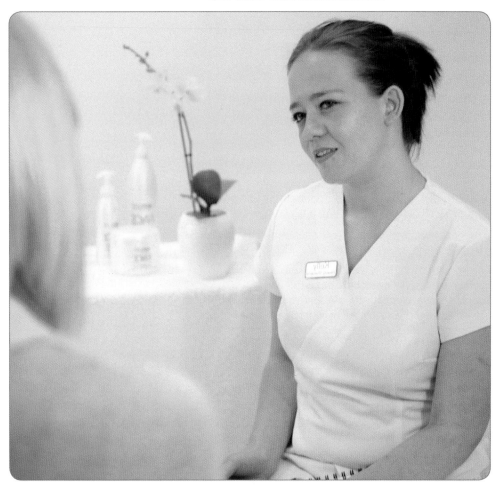

Carrying out a client consultation

Planning and preparing your treatment will always involve a **client consultation**. Until you have talked to the client about why she has come to the salon for a facial and assessed her skin type and any problems, it will not be possible for you to decide which products and techniques to use on your client. Client consultation involves the following three methods:

- questioning and recording information
- visual analysis
- manual analysis – this is when you feel the smoothness, softness, firmness and hydration of the client's skin.

Questioning

Clients will want facials for many different reasons. Depending on their reasons, this will help to shape the type of facial that should be offered to them and the techniques used.

For relaxation and a feeling of well-being

To add moisture to dry or dehydrated skin

Reasons why a client might want a facial

To help clear spots and **blemishes**

To reduce the oil on greasy skin

Reasons for a facial treatment

It is therefore very important that you ask the client about her wishes and needs from the facial and listen and respond carefully. Sitting down to talk with the client about what she wants will also give you the opportunity to ask her about her skin and any problem areas, as well as the skin care routine that she follows at home.

Top tip ✓

At first you will watch and learn from the therapist while she is carrying out a consultation. Eventually you will have gained enough experience to carry out the consultation yourself under the supervision of the therapist.

FACIAL CONSULTATION CARD

DATE 12/02/10

CLIENT'S NAME Miss Nadia Shah

ADDRESS 14 Willow Crescent, Newtown N01 3JA

DATE OF BIRTH 26/08/78

TELEPHONE NUMBER (H) 0208 976 1133

(W) 0207 612 1060

CONDITION OF SKIN ON INSPECTION

Clear complexion, fine lines around the eyes, a few broken capillaries on cheek area. Feels slightly dry.

CONTRA-INDICATIONS/CONDITIONS

No contra-indications. Comedones around nose and chin.

PRODUCTS USED

Nourishing Nature's range for dry skin.

HOMECARE ADVICE

Drink more water to rehydrate the skin.
Use sunscreen and exfoliate weekly.

PRODUCT SALES

Nourishing Nature's trial pack for dry skin.

COMMENTS

Client was very relaxed and pleased with how her skin felt. Has re-booked for a month's time.

CLIENT SIGNATURE

RECORD OF TREATMENTS

DATE	TREATMENT	THERAPIST
12/02/10	Facial	Sarah Walker

A typical consultation card for a facial treatment

While you question the client, you need to start filling in a **client consultation** card with the information that the client gives you. An example of a consultation card for a facial skin care treatment is shown above. Some of the information will be filled in later, after you have studied the skin, and some when you have completed the treatment, but all of the information you need is included in the diagram on page 226 for easy reference. Have a look at Unit B1 Prepare and maintain salon treatment work areas to refresh your memory about why it is important to record the information.

≫ Get up and go!

Design a simple flow chart showing the stages of the consultation that you can use to jog your memory. Display it on a postcard so that it will fit on your trolley next to you. Remember to laminate it so that you protect it from spills and splashes.

Consult, plan and prepare for treatments with clients [4]

Recording information

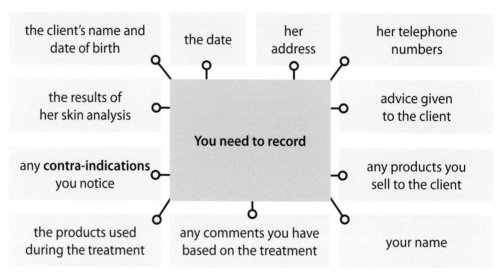

Information you need to record for a facial skin care treatment

> ✓ **Top tips**
>
> - Name – there could be two clients with the same surname, so to avoid confusion, make sure you always write down both the client's first name and surname.
> - Address – remember to include the postcode.
> - Telephone number – one telephone number is not enough. If you need to call a client at short notice to tell her that you have to cancel her appointment and you have her home phone number but she is at work, you will not be able to get in touch, so always ask for a home number and a work or mobile number.
> - Date of birth – you may need to find out your client's date of birth, as if she is under the age of 16 a parent or guardian must be present throughout the treatment. Also the parent or guardian must sign the consultation to agree for the treatment to go ahead – this is called giving consent.

Visual analysis

After talking to the client and noting down the information you need to record, you then need to study the client's skin visually. This should be done in good light so that you are able to see the skin's condition and texture and includes finding out about:

- skin type
- skin condition
- contra-indications.

Skin types and conditions

Deciding on a client's skin type is essential before you can decide on the best treatment for her skin. There are four main skin types, and each of the four skin types may also have other characteristics that are important for you to note.

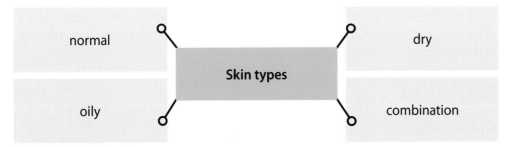

The four main skin types

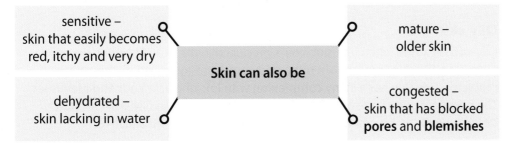

Characteristics that each of the four skin types may display

> **» Get up and go!**
>
> Make some key cards to help you remember the different types of skin and the characteristics of each. Write 'normal skin' on one card, then turn it over and write a description of the characteristics of normal skin on the back. Make a card like this for each of the skin types. You can use these to test each other on skin types and conditions.

> **? Memory jogger**
>
> 1 What are the three types of consultation techniques?
> 2 List four pieces of information that you would need to record when carrying out a consultation.
> 3 Why is it important to ask a client about her wishes?

Consult, plan and prepare for treatments with clients (5)

Deciding on a client's skin type is not always a simple process – it can take several years to master each part of a facial treatment and become an expert. However, for Level 1 only background knowledge of the basics is required. Let's take a closer look at skin types.

Skin types

Normal skin

Normal skin is a rare skin type. It is usually found in children and young clients. It is smooth and clear with no **blemishes**. It feels soft to touch and has very tiny **pores** that are difficult to see. This type of skin needs lots of gentle care to keep it normal.

Oily skin

Oily skin is caused when too much oil is produced in the skin. Although we need oil to keep the skin smooth, when the body produces too much oil this causes problems. Oily skin has a shiny **complexion** with lots of blackheads and blemishes. The **pores** are quite large and the skin can be quite thick. An oily skin can start or become worse as a teenager, when puberty hormones are most active.

Dry skin

Dry skin is lacking in oil and may flake and chap easily. It can feel tight after washing, especially if soap is used. Dry skin absorbs creams and lotions quickly, and can become lined and wrinkled early (especially around the eyes) unless it is **moisturised** well. Poor diet or **dehydration** can cause dry skin or make it worse.

Combination skin

Combination skin is made up of two skin types. These types vary but the most common is normal or dry skin on the cheek area, and an oily part on the nose and chin, and across the forehead (known as the T-zone). The oily T-zone shows up as a shiny nose, chin and forehead with blackheads.

 Get up and go!

What skin type are you?

Take a close look at your skin in the mirror. Use a good light and decide what skin type you have.

Next, pair up with a friend and inspect each other's skin. Did you both agree on the skin type?

Contra-indications

A **contra-indication** is a condition that makes or could make a client unsuitable for a treatment. At Level 1 you are not responsible for deciding whether or not a client has a contra-indication, but you must be aware of them and be able to recognise the signs so that you can tell a senior therapist if you notice anything unusual.

Whatever level of experience therapists have, they are not qualified to diagnose medical conditions. Quite often during your treatments you may have an idea of what medical condition a client may have, but you must refer them to their GP. You must also make sure that you do not cause the client alarm or embarrassment by talking loudly about a contra-indication so that other people may hear or in a way that may worry the client.

Working around contra-indications

Some contra-indications can be worked around and you can adapt your treatment in line with the client's needs. Usually you will avoid the area that must not be worked on, but sometimes it is difficult to do this and so you may need to:

- cover the area with a plaster
- cover the area with barrier cream.

Contra-indications that may be worked around include:

- non-infectious conditions
- non-recent scar tissue (over six months old)
- mild bruising
- grazes or small cuts.

Skin disorders that may restrict treatment include:

- healed **eczema** – this will present as very dry and parched skin and can quite often look very lined
- psoriasis – this is scaly flakes of skin, quite often red and inflamed. It is best to completely avoid these areas as the products and procedures could cause further inflammation
- redness – adapt your methods, for example use gentle products and don't carry out stimulating massage movements
- bruising – work around the bruising so that you don't cause pain to the client
- skin irritation – it is recommended that you postpone the treatment until the irritation goes as it could be a sign of an allergy.

Consult, plan and prepare for treatments with clients [6]

Total contra-indications

Some **contra-indications** could be made worse by treatment or could be infectious and spread to you and your other clients. These are called total contra-indications. You must never treat a client who has a total contra-indication.

You will need to look out for:

- splits or blisters around the nose and mouth that could be a cold sore
- bloodshot and watery eyes that could be an allergy or **conjunctivitis**
- extremely red skin – it could be a sign of an allergy or an injury
- swelling or lumps – it could just be bruising but could also be something much more serious that needs to be checked by a GP.

The following photos should help you to know what to look out for when you check a client's skin for contra-indications.

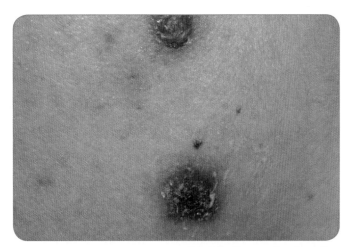

Skin infections such as impetigo

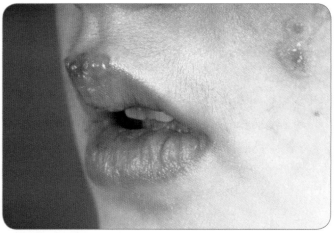

Cold sores

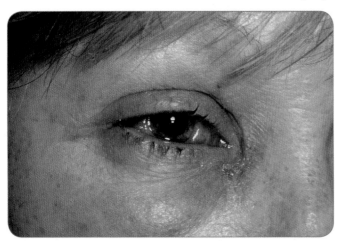

Conjunctivitis

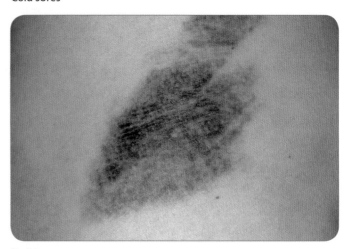

Bruising

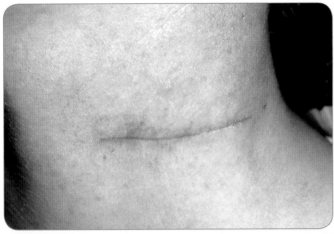

Scar tissue less than six months old

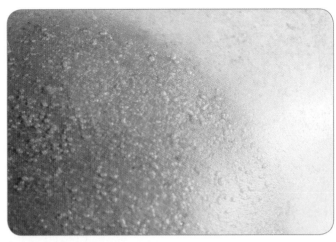

Recent sunburn

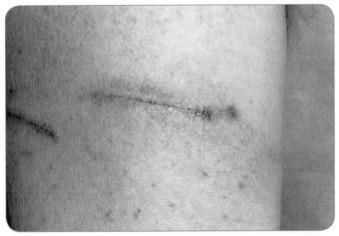

Cuts and grazes

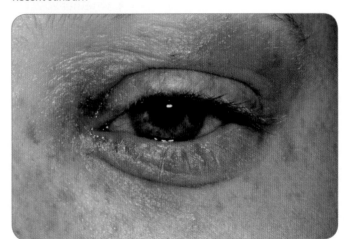

Eczema

Allergies

Some clients may be allergic to certain ingredients contained in products. You should always ask your client if she has any known **allergies** and check the list of ingredients on the label of the products you are planning to use.

It may be that you check for allergies beforehand but a client nevertheless reacts badly to a product by showing one of these signs: itching, tightness, blistering, watery eyes, excess sweating, swelling or redness. If this happens you must take steps to remove the product immediately and tell your supervisor, who will advise you and the client on what should be done. She may be advised to bathe the area with cool water and see her GP.

 Top tip

If you notice anything unusual on the skin, always ask your tutor or senior therapist to check for you before you start the treatment.

Consult, plan and prepare for treatments with clients (7)

Adapting your manner for different clients

Although your manner must always be professional, your consultation with your client gives you the opportunity to find out what your client is like. Remember that the conversation and personality that one client may enjoy, another may not. Find out:

- what your client likes and does not like
- what your client's personality is like; for example, shy or extrovert
- whether your client is talkative or quiet.

As an assistant therapist you do not yet have the client experience that more qualified therapists have and so it is important that you try to develop people skills and learn how and when you need to adapt your body language, speech and manner. Use this consultation time to learn about the client so that you can adapt your style of communication as well as the treatment.

Preparing the client

Once you have finished the **client consultation**, you need to get the client ready for her facial treatment.

1 Ask the client to remove any jewellery she is wearing and ask her to store it safely.

2 Ask the client to remove the clothes from her top half, and take them and hang them up. If she has to go to a treatment cubicle to change, you will need to give her a gown to wear to prevent any embarrassment.

3 Help the client on to the couch. Remove the gown and cover the client with the blankets or towels, and ask her if she is warm and comfortable.

4 Protect the client's hair with a headband. Tuck either tissue or couch roll under the headband to keep it as clean as possible. Place a medium-sized towel across the client's chest, then slip her bra straps down over her upper arms and tuck the towel over and under the straps, to protect them from the products.

 Top tip

If a client removes her jewellery and does place it in a dish, the jewellery dish should then be placed on top of the trolley so that the client is able to see it at all times. This is for security reasons and it also acts as a memory jogger, so that the client does not forget her jewellery when she leaves.

Consulting, planning and preparing for treatments with clients: a checklist

1 Have you prepared yourself and checked your personal presentation?

2 Have you set up your workplace and checked that you have what you need and that your equipment and tools are organised, easy to reach and properly sterilised or disinfected?

3 Have you removed your watch and jewellery?

4 Have you washed your hands?

5 Have you carried out the consultation?

6 Have you assessed the condition of your client's skin?

7 Have you checked for **contra-indications**?

8 Have you asked the client to remove her jewellery?

9 Have you asked the client to remove the clothes from her top half, helped her on to the couch, covered her, protected her hair and bra straps and checked if she is warm and comfortable?

If so, you are ready to begin the facial treatment.

 Salon life

Deepak started to cleanse the skin of his client but she started to wriggle and complained that it was stinging a bit. Deepak thought that this would be fine and they agreed he would carry on, so he then toned the skin, but he could see the skin getting redder and redder and his client's lips then began to swell too. His supervisor had popped out for a ten-minute break to get a bite to eat, so he did not have anyone to ask what to do. He checked the record card and there was no information to say that his client had an allergy, so he removed the cleanser and toner that he had used with cool water and tried to calm the reaction with different products. The condition got worse and by the time his supervisor returned the client's face was very red and swollen and his supervisor was horrified.

Was it Deepak's fault?

What could Deepak have done to lessen the problem?

What could you do to prevent this happening to you?

? **Memory jogger**

1 List three contra-indications that you could work around.

2 List three contra-indications that will prevent you carrying out the treatment.

3 List the steps you need to take to prepare your client.

4 List three signs of an allergy.

5 How do you protect a contra-indication that you can work around?

Carry out facial treatments [1]

A facial should be relaxing and enjoyable for the client, as well as being beneficial to her skin. Learning about carrying out a facial involves learning about several smaller treatments that are carried out to:

- deep clean the **pores**
- nourish and **rehydrate** the skin
- relax the muscles
- improve the circulation
- brighten the **complexion**.

After a facial, the client should feel relaxed and her skin should glow.

Step-by-step facial

There are many steps involved in a facial skin care treatment. Before we go into them in detail, it will help to look at this summary so that the procedure is clear.

Start

1 Preparation and consultation	2 Check for contra-indications	3 Eye make-up removal
6 Tone and refresh	5 Second cleanse	4 First cleanse
7 Full skin inspection	8 Exfoliate, steam and comedone removal	9 Massage
12 Soften and smooth	11 Tone and refresh	10 Face mask

Finish

Summary of steps in a facial treatment

Top tip

Throughout the facial, explain what you are doing and why. This will reassure the client and help her to relax and enjoy it.

Make-up removal

When your client is prepared for her facial and comfortably positioned on the couch, the first thing you need to do is to remove any make-up that she might be wearing. This is shown on page 238.

 Top tip

You may need to repeat the eye make-up removal process for very heavy or waterproof make-up.

Cleansing

Your next step is to cleanse the client's face. Choose an appropriate cleanser for the client – look back at page 222 to remind yourself of the different types of cleansers available.

The cleansing routine is carried out with massage movements. Massage has three main movements.

- **Effleurage:** this is a gentle stroking movement used at the beginning or end of the treatment or to join up other movements. It has a soothing and relaxing effect. This is the technique used for cleansing.
- **Petrissage:** these movements are circular or kneading movements. The hands, thumbs or fingertips are used to apply pressure to the muscles by lifting, rolling and pushing.
- **Tapotement:** this is a more stimulating movement in which the fingers, sides or palms of the hands produce light tapping, quick pinching or gentle slapping movements.

For Level 1, it is not necessary for you to follow a set massage routine using all the movements. However, it is important to carry out some sort of pattern that is relaxing to the client. The photos on pages 238–242 illustrate a simple cleansing routine for you to follow.

All movements are done lightly and your hands must never leave the client's skin.

Tone and refresh

After cleansing the client's skin twice, you then need to refresh her skin and remove the last traces of cleanser using a toning lotion. This is shown on page 243.

 Top tip

Remember that you will have to write down the products you use on the client's face on her record card.

Carry out facial treatments (2)

Step-by-step facial

Full skin inspection

When your client's skin is completely clean, dry and grease-free, your senior therapist will carry out a thorough skin inspection under the magnifying lamp. It is only now when the skin is absolutely clean that you and your senior therapist will be able to see the true skin type, any disorders and make a final check for any **contra-indications**. You will then also be able to plan the rest of your facial deciding:

- on the products to be used
- on the type of face mask
- whether you need to slightly change your treatment plan.

When carrying out the skin inspection, make notes on the record card.

Skin disorders and contra-indications

Look out for signs of these, which were covered on pages 229–231.

Skin colour • Does it have a healthy glow? • Are there areas of redness that could suggest sensitivity? • Is the skin tanned or is it a yellowy colour?	**The eyes** • Are there laughter lines around the eyes? • Are there dark circles or puffiness around or under the eyes?
Skin texture Touch the skin. How does it feel? • Soft or rough? • Dry or oily? • Flaky or smooth? • Thin or thick? • Firm or loose?	**Skin and muscle tone** • Is the skin young and firm with good muscle tone and tight skin? • Is the skin around the eyes and mouth loose with lines and wrinkles? • Are there frown lines on the forehead?
The T-zone • Is the T-zone shiny with blackheads, spots and open **pores**?	**Client information** Ask the client: • what products she uses on her skin • what her normal skincare routine is.

What to look for during a full skin inspection

Exfoliate, steam and comedone removal, and massage

The next steps in the facial treatment are exfoliation, steaming and comedone extraction, and massage, which will all be carried out by a senior therapist.

Massage is a very skilful part of the facial treatment and can take a long time to master, so make sure that you watch the senior therapist carefully. As you become more skilled at your treatment, you may be allowed to carry out part of the massage.

>> **Get up and go!**

Practise some massage movements on another therapist so that she can give you feedback on how to improve.

Face mask

When the senior therapist has completed the massage, you will then apply the face mask. Before applying the face mask, make sure that your client's skin is free of oils and creams. Then choose a pre-prepared, non-setting mask to suit your client's skin type.

Soften and smooth

The final stage of the facial treatment is applying moisturiser to the client's skin. When you have finished, leave the client to relax for a couple of minutes, and go and wash your hands. Then offer your client a mirror, so that she can check her **complexion**.

Finishing touches

When you have finished the facial treatment, you must:

- ask your client how she feels and if she is pleased with her treatment
- give your client homecare advice (see pages 246–247)
- check the finished result with the senior therapist
- check the time, to make sure that the treatment was cost-effective and carried out within an acceptable time (see page 320–321)
- make sure that the workplace is left tidy, clean and ready for further treatments.

Remember to complete the client's record card with as much information as possible on the products you used, the homecare advice you gave her on how to improve the condition of her skin and when to return for another salon treatment, your comments on how you and the client thought the treatment went, and the date, the type of facial and your name.

Top tips

- It is very important to check that every trace of the mask is removed – make sure that no mask remains anywhere on the skin. Check behind the ears and under the chin.
- Always follow the manufacturer's instructions when using beauty products. The instructions should have information about:
  - how to use the product
  - how long to leave it on the skin
  - how to store it
  - how to use it safely.

≫ Get up and go!

Design a client feedback sheet that you can use to ask clients how they felt about their facial treatment.

Discuss the feedback with the rest of your class and your tutor.

? Memory jogger

1 At what stage in the facial do you apply the face mask?
2 Why is it important to write down on the record card all of the products that you use during a facial?
3 When do you give the client homecare advice?
4 Where on the face would the oily section usually be found with a combination skin type?
5 What would the texture of the skin feel like on a client with mature skin?
6 Why must the skin be completely clean and free of make-up before carrying out a full skin inspection?

Carry out facial treatments (3)

Step-by-step facial

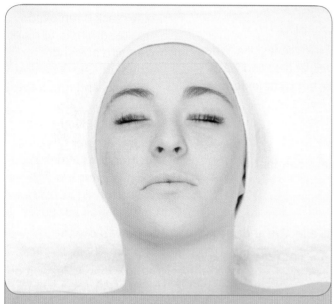

1   Make sure the client is prepared for her facial.

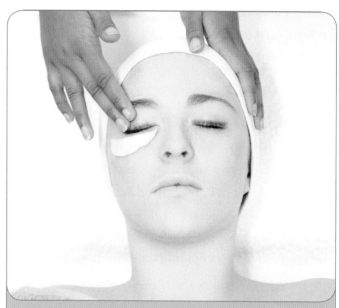

2   Place half moons under the bottom lashes and ask client to close her eyes. Squeeze a small amount of eye make-up remover on to a spatula. Dip your index finger into the cleanser and gently rub on and around the eye in a circular movement.

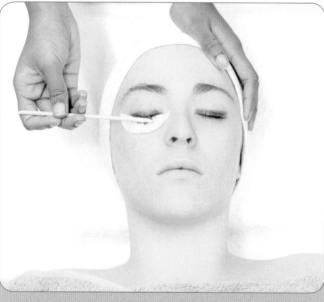

3   Using a covered orange stick, use gentle downward strokes until the eye and lashes are free from make-up and cleanser. Repeat on the other eye. Then ask the client to open her eyes so that you can clean underneath them.

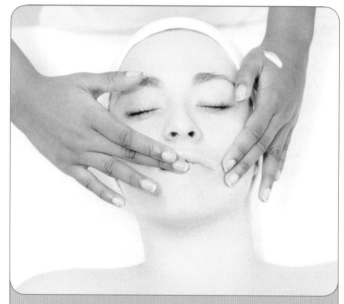

4   Gently rub some cleanser on to the lips. Hold on one side of the mouth for support, then wipe the make-up away with the other hand using damp cotton wool. Then hold the other side of the mouth, and repeat.

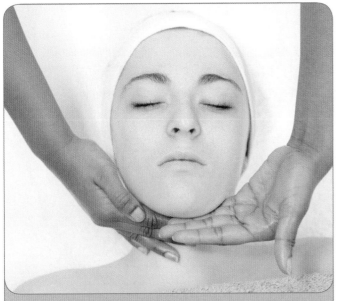

5   Squeeze a small amount of cleanser into the palm of your hands, then put your hands together so that you have the cleanser in both hands. Gently press your hands over the face and neck of your client, to coat her skin in cleanser.

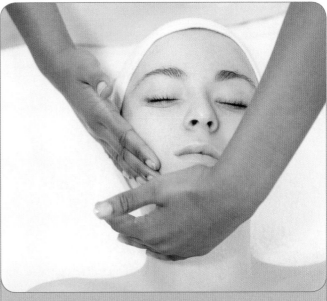

6   Using gentle, upward **effleurage** strokes, distribute the cleanser evenly over the face.

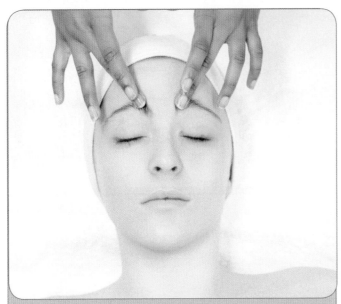

7   Following the direction of the brows, gently circle the eyes with the middle fingers to distribute the cleanser around the eyes.

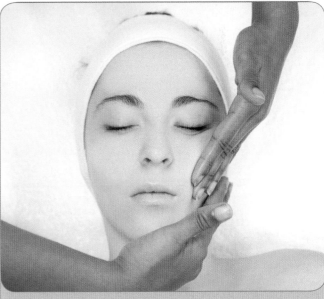

8   Use gentle upward effleurage strokes to spread the cleanser over the cheeks.

Carry out facial treatments [4]

Step-by-step facial

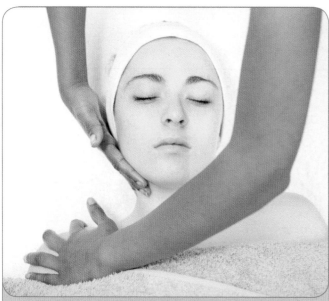

9 Using light movements, apply eight upward strokes to the client's shoulders, chest area and neck with the palms of your hands. Start with the left side and gradually work to the right side. Then repeat, this time working from the right side to the left side.

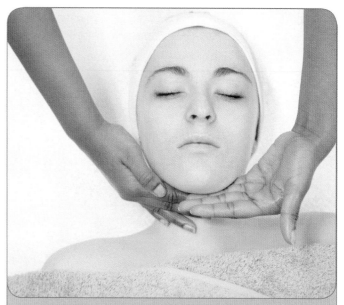

10 Apply eight upward strokes to the client's neck with the palms of your hands. Start with the left side and gradually work to the right side. Then repeat, this time working from the right side to the left side.

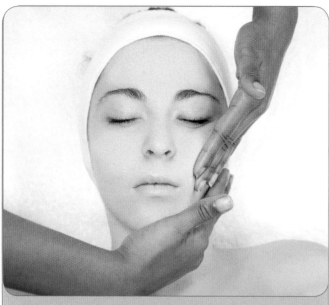

11 Using the palms of the hands, slide to the left cheek and stroke upwards eight times.

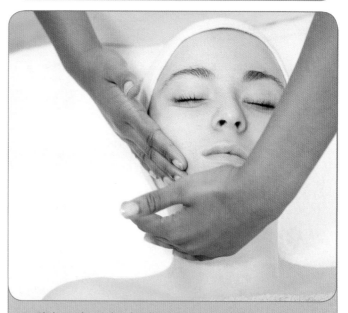

12 Slide to the right cheek and stroke upwards eight times.

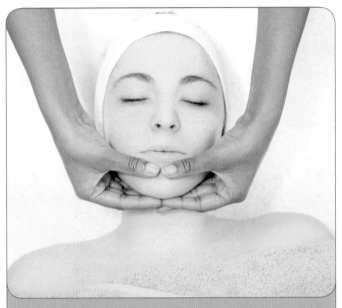

13 Slide to the chin and carry out upward thumb circles eight times.

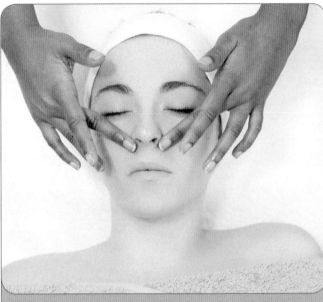

14 Using middle or index fingers, circle eight times under and around the sides of the nose.

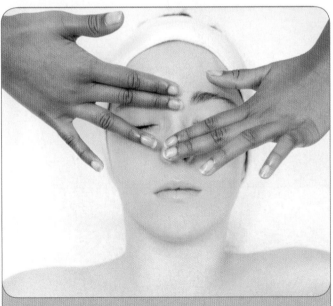

15 Slide up to the bridge of the nose and stroke upwards four times.

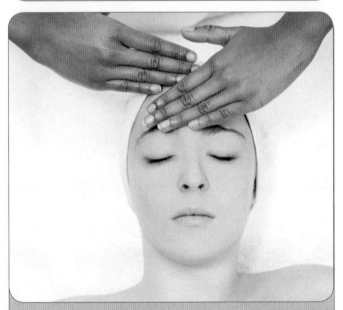

16 Slide up to the forehead and stroke upwards eight times, moving from the left to the right and then back again.

Carry out facial treatments (5)

Step-by-step facial

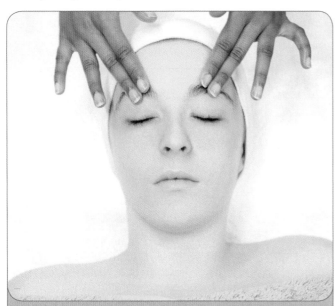

17 Slide your hands to the middle of the forehead and circle the eyes gently four times in the direction of growth of the eyebrow. Slide to the temples and apply gentle pressure to complete the cleansing routine.

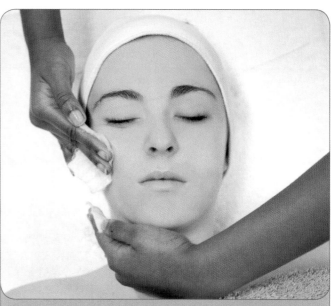

18 Take two damp cotton wool squares and wrap them around your first two fingers, and use them to remove the cleanser, which has now mixed with the dirt and face make-up. Use exactly the same strokes as for the cleansing routine (steps 9 to 17).

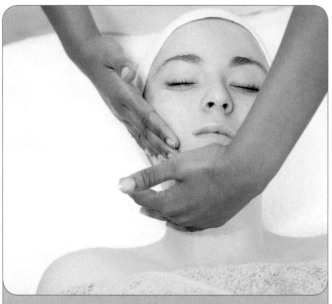

19 Carry out a second cleanse by repeating steps 5 to 19.

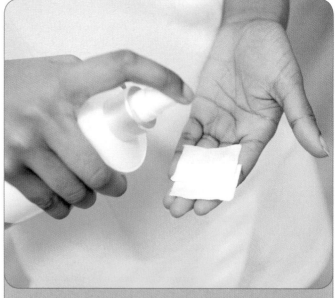

20 Take two more damp cotton wool squares and soak them in toning lotion.

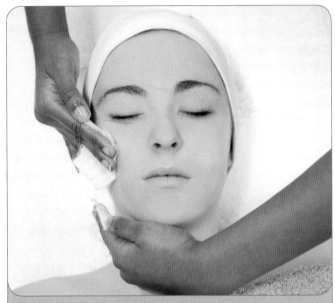

21 Wrap the cotton wool around your fingers and repeat the cleaning routine, using the toner on the cotton wool instead. This will tone the skin and remove the last traces of cleanser.

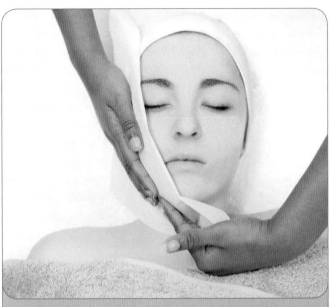

22 Using a split tissue, blot the toning lotion. Tone the skin a second time.

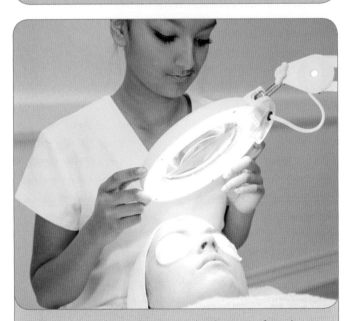

23 Carry out a skin inspection under the magnifying lamp.

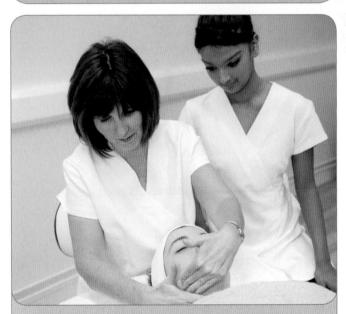

24 The senior therapist will carry out a skin exfoliating treatment, steam and comedone extraction. Tone and blot the skin by repeating steps 21 and 22. The senior therapist will then massage the client's face, neck and shoulders. The massage should last about 15–20 minutes.

Carry out facial treatments (6)

Step-by-step facial

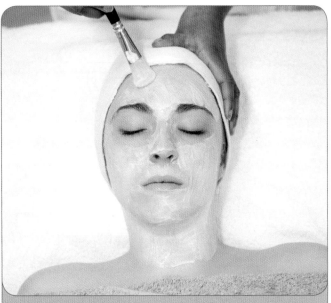

25 Place enough mask in a bowl to coat all your client's face and neck. Using a mask brush and starting at the neck, apply the mask to the skin and move upwards evenly in smooth strokes, finishing with the forehead. Avoid the lips, eyes, nostrils and hairline.

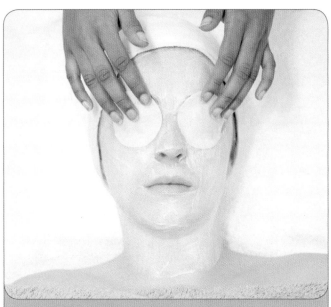

26 After the face mask has been applied, place eye circles over your client's eyes, then leave her to rest and relax for about 10 minutes, depending on the manufacturer's instructions.

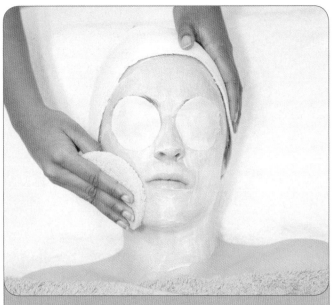

27 After 10 minutes remove the eye pads and press damp sponges over the mask, allowing the water to soak in. Starting at the neck and working up over the cheeks on to the nose and forehead, remove all the face mask with firm upward strokes.

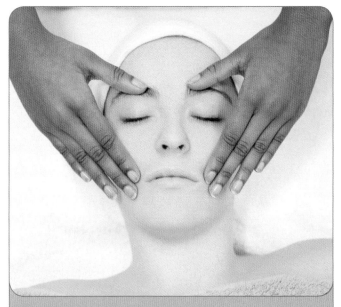

28 Tone and blot the skin and apply moisturiser for the client's skin type using the same massage routine to apply the moisturiser as you did for the cleanser. Blot the skin if there is too much moisturiser on it.

Making sure your client enjoys her facial

A facial should be an enjoyable and relaxing treatment for your client, but this could be spoiled if you are careless or disorganised. A client may not enjoy a facial if the therapist:

- has offensive body odour or bad breath or smells of tobacco
- harms or scratches the skin with jewellery, watches or nails that are too long
- massages the skin excessively or roughly
- gets facial creams or products into the client's eyes
- breathes into the client's face
- is not hygienic or careful enough
- removes cream carelessly and incorrectly, leaving a greasy film behind the ears, under the chin or in other areas
- does not permit the client to relax, either by talking too much or being tense while giving the treatment
- is disorganised and needs to leave the client to go and fetch materials and products
- has heavy, rough or cold hands.

Take care to avoid these mistakes!

Male facials

More men are having facial treatments than ever before. It is now seen as acceptable for men to visit salons to have treatments, and there are ranges of skin care products available in shops and salons that are targeted at the male skin care market. This has become a very profitable business.

 Salon life

During a consultation, Petra asked her client what she hoped to gain from her facial. The client said that she had a big dinner party that evening and wanted to go out feeling like a 'new woman'. The client said that her skin was dry and flaky, and that her make-up wouldn't go on very smoothly. The client hoped that Petra would be able to improve the texture of her skin, so that her make-up would look great for the party.

It was obvious to Petra that the client had not been advised as to what a facial is, and therefore had her heart set on:

- a treatment for dry flaky skin
- being able to apply great make-up for her dinner party.
1 How could Petra explain the purpose of a facial to her client?
2 What other choices could Petra give her client?

Write down or discuss how you would deal with these problems.

 Top tip

Although you want to make sure that your client is enjoying her treatment by asking her how it feels or if she is comfortable, asking her too many times during the facial can ruin the atmosphere of the treatment and mean that it will not be as relaxing for her. Try not to question her more than a couple of times.

Get up and go!

Visit some local salons and find out about the male skin care treatments on offer. How do they differ from a female skin care treatment?

Provide aftercare advice

So that the beneficial effects of the facial treatment lasts, it is important to give the client some advice after the treatment.

You should advise your client that the recommended interval between facial treatments is one month in order to keep the skin in great condition. This also gives your client the opportunity to book a further appointment with the salon.

The facial treatment has given your client's skin a boost. After the treatment, her skin will enjoy better circulation and a softer texture, and should be the cleanest it has been for a while. It is therefore important to give your client follow-up advice, so that she can experience the long-term benefits of her treatment. The table below details the follow-up advice that you should give.

Follow-up advice	Reasons for advice
Leave the skin alone for the next 12 hours – it is not even necessary to cleanse it that night	The skin has had an hour-long treatment to deep cleanse and stimulate it, so it is best to allow time for the skin to relax and the salon products to work
Do not apply make-up for 12 hours, if possible	Make-up could clog the skin **pores** and make the skin dirty again before it has had a chance to gain the full benefits of the treatment
Avoid touching the skin	Touching the skin will make it dirty and undo the good work of the facial
Have a monthly facial, if possible	The skin takes about a month to renew its layers, so a regular facial will keep it in great condition
Cleanse, tone and **moisturise**, both morning and evening	This will keep the skin and pores clean and the skin soft
Wear a good moisturiser under make-up and in cold and windy weather	A good moisturiser will protect the skin from getting clogged with make-up and drying out in bad weather
Drink plenty of water and eat a healthy diet with lots of fruit and fresh vegetables	Water will help to **rehydrate** dry skin and a good diet will improve the condition of all skin types
Get plenty of sleep	When we sleep, the skin has a chance to repair itself
Try not to touch or squeeze blackheads and spots	You could make the problem worse and damage the skin
Always protect skin in the sun by using a cream containing a UV-filter (at least SPF 15)	The sun can age and dry out skin

 Top tip

Look back at the Anatomy and physiology section in this book and refresh your memory on tips for healthy skin that you can pass on to your client.

Contra-actions

It is also helpful to give the client information on possible **contra-actions**. These are unwanted reactions that could occur, during or after a facial skin care treatment. If these happen during the treatment, the treatment may need to be stopped mid-way through and steps taken to prevent it happening again in the future. If there are no problems during the treatment, you nevertheless need to make the client aware of possible contra-actions in case she experiences them after leaving the salon.

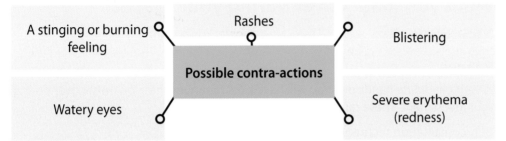

A stinging or burning feeling

Rashes

Blistering

Possible contra-actions

Watery eyes

Severe erythema (redness)

Possible contra-actions to a facial skin care treatment

? Memory jogger

1 Give six points of follow-up advice and the reasons for them.
2 List three possible contra-indications that the client should be aware of before she leaves the salon.

Getting ready for assessment

Evidence requirements

You will be observed by your assessor on at least three occasions, each involving a different client.

What you must cover during your practical assessments

Ranges

In your candidate handbook you will have a list of ranges that you must cover during your assessment. These ranges cover:

1 consultation techniques

2 skin types

3 client preparation

4 facial products

5 advice.

It is good practice to cover as many ranges as possible during each assessment. This will prevent you having to take too many additional assessments because there are many ranges that you have not managed to cover.

Performance criteria

What you must demonstrate during a practical observation by your tutor:

- preparation for facials
- a skin analysis
- good communication skills
- basic facial skin care treatment using:
  - cleansers, toners, moisturisers and eye make-up remover
  - tools, equipment and consumables
  - skin care products
  - eye products
- checking the client is happy with the facial skin care treatment
- giving aftercare advice to the client
- leaving the work area in a suitable condition.

Throughout your observations you will also need to make sure that you pay attention to health, safety and hygiene throughout, as well as presenting yourself well, so read through Unit G20 Make sure your own actions reduce risks to health and safety before any practical assessment just to refresh your memory.

Carrying out a practical treatment using unhygienic tools, or without carrying out a risk assessment of your work area to avoid accidents happening, will mean that you are not safe to do a treatment and therefore could mean that you do not pass your assessment.

What you must know

In order to pass this unit, you will need to gather evidence during the teaching and learning of this unit before your assessor observes your practical performance. You will gather this during class work and further study and will probably file it in a portfolio of evidence. This evidence will also be signed off in your candidate handbook which you will be given by your assessor. This will be an official record to show that you have covered what you need to.

 Salon life

The senior therapist asked Maz to carry out the cleansing routine on a new client. During the questioning, Maz worked out that the client was 40 years old, but when Maz removed all of the make-up she was quite shocked to see that the client's skin was very yellow and thick and the lines on the face were so much deeper than other mature clients she had treated that actually the client looked more like 60.

While Maz was doing the cleansing routine the client looked up at Maz and complimented her on her complexion, she then asked her where she had got her tan. Maz told her that she sits out in her garden at weekends in the summer and visits the local tanning salon in the winter.

The client then gave Maz a lecture on the dangers of sunbathing and sunbeds and told her that if she continued her skin would look like hers. Maz was shocked!

Find out about the effects of the sun and sunbeds on the skin.

How can Maz learn from her client?

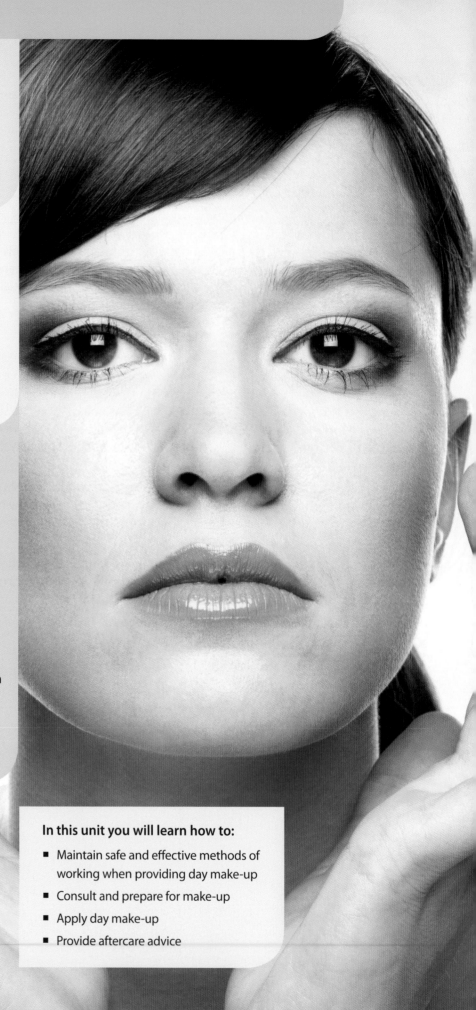

UNIT B3

Assist with day make-up

Make-up can be considered an art form as it allows you to combine imagination and creative thinking to create all kinds of looks using different colour combinations, techniques and styles. There are no set rules other than that you should enhance the client's natural features and give her a look that gives her confidence in her appearance.

In this unit you will learn about safe and hygienic methods of application, carrying out client consultations, make-up application and giving aftercare advice. You will develop practical skills to assist in make-up application while learning about the wide range of make-up products and the use of tools such as brushes, applicators and mixing palettes.

In this unit you will learn how to:

- Maintain safe and effective methods of working when providing day make-up
- Consult and prepare for make-up
- Apply day make-up
- Provide aftercare advice

Here are some key terms you may meet in this unit:

Consultation –
a discussion, talk

Lanolin –
a natural oil that comes
from sheep's wool

Anti-bacterial –
something that cuts down
the spread of germs and
infections

Semi-reclining –
lying down but not
completely flat

Allergens –
things that can cause
unwanted allergic
reactions

Psoriasis –
a skin condition consisting
of itchy, dry red patches

Erythema –
abnormal redness
of the skin

Acetone –
a flammable substance
used in nail polish

Dry skin –
skin that is lacking in oil
and may flake and
chap easily

Stipple –
pressing and rolling
action

Dermatitis –
inflammation of
the skin

Combination skin –
skin that is usually made up
of normal and dry skin on the
cheeks and oily skin on the
nose and forehead

Normal skin –
skin that is smooth
with no blemishes

Oily skin –
skin that is shiny with
quite large pores

T-zone –
the nose, chin and forehead,
which can be oily

Maintain safe and effective methods of working when providing day make-up [1]

Make-up is no different to any other treatment in a salon. Safety, hygiene and preparation are just as important as they would be for facials or any other treatment.

When you are applying your make-up on yourself at home, it is unlikely that you would think about whether you have used techniques and products that are safe and hygienic. However, when applying make-up on a client, the habits and methods you use at home would probably not be acceptable in the salon.

The work area

Whether you are carrying out your make-up application on a couch or make-up chair, your tutor/assessor will guide you in how to set up your work area and the preparation of the correct products, tools and equipment necessary in the first instance. However, there are essential things that will be required in order to carry out the make-up treatment effectively and these products, tools and equipment are covered on pages 256–257.

The most important requirements are that your set-up is:

- organised – nothing forgotten, all equipment and tools on a trolley, set up in the order of when it will be used
- easy to reach – you will not have to overstretch to reach it or walk across the room
- hygienic – everything is cleaned, disinfected and sterilised, and your couch or chair has a protective cover.

It is very important to be organised with everything to hand as it can be very off-putting to the client if the therapist keeps leaving her to go and fetch something that has been forgotten.

Sterilisation and cleaning of make-up tools and equipment

Where possible you should use disposable applicators for applying make-up as this is the most hygienic method. Make-up brushes should be washed in warm soapy water and left to dry naturally before placing in an ultraviolet cabinet (see Unit G20, pages 26–27 for more details on sterilisation and cleaning methods).

Top tip ✓

It is very easy to spread germs from one client to another by using dirty brushes and towels, putting fingers in pots or setting up on a dirty work surface. This is why sterilisation and hygiene procedures are so important.

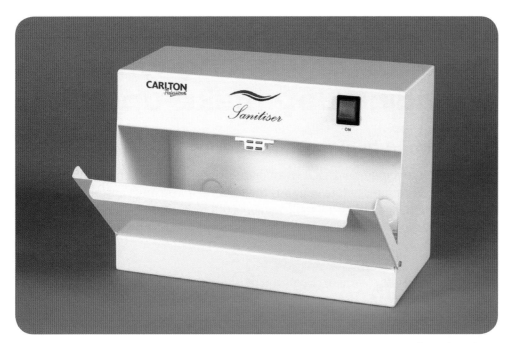

Ultraviolet cabinet

All make-up products should be removed from their containers using a disposable spatula or orange stick and placed on a clean make-up palette.

After use the make-up palette should be cleaned with warm soapy water and then wiped over with disinfectant solution.

Lip and eye pencils should be sharpened before use on each client as this means that they have a fresh and sterile surface.

Make-up sponges should be thrown away after use as it is very difficult to clean them thoroughly. If they are reused they should be washed with warm soapy water and left to dry naturally before placing in an ultraviolet cabinet.

✓ Top tip

Don't blow on make-up brushes to remove loose make-up powder before use, as this will make them unhygienic. Instead, shake the loose powder off on to a clean tissue.

≫ Get up and go!

Make a poster with pictures of your make-up tools and equipment showing how you need to clean, disinfect or sterilise them.

? Memory jogger

1 How do you protect your couch or make-up chair?
2 Why should lip and eye pencils be sharpened before use on each client?
3 What is the best way to clean make-up brushes?
4 How should you remove products from their containers?

Maintain safe and effective methods of working when providing day make-up (2)

Maintaining hygiene throughout

It is important to remember that it is not enough to simply follow good hygiene and preparation procedures before you start the treatment. You must ensure that the tools, equipment and yourself remain hygienic throughout the treatment too. (See Unit G20, pages 26–27 for more information on sterilisation and preventing cross-infection.)

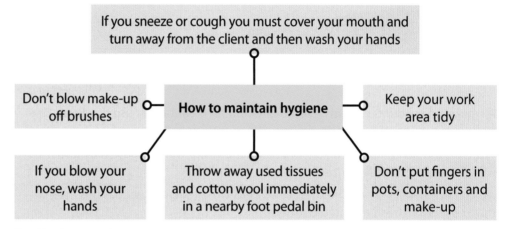

If you sneeze or cough you must cover your mouth and turn away from the client and then wash your hands

Don't blow make-up off brushes

How to maintain hygiene

Keep your work area tidy

If you blow your nose, wash your hands

Throw away used tissues and cotton wool immediately in a nearby foot pedal bin

Don't put fingers in pots, containers and make-up

Good hygiene practices

Leaving the work area clean and tidy

If you don't leave your work area clean and tidy it will not be in a fit condition to be used by the next therapist who wishes to carry out another treatment. It goes without saying that a client should not be brought into an untidy and dirty room as this will create a bad impression and could lose the salon customers.

If you have used up equipment and not replaced it, or left the room untidy, the next therapist to use the room will look disorganised and the client may lose confidence in her even though it is not her fault.

Even after you have finished the treatment and your client has left, hygiene and safety are still important. It is essential that you clear away all of your tools and equipment and that you leave your work area clean and tidy. This includes:

- wiping over trolleys, couches, bins and stools with disinfectant
- washing your brushes and palette
- putting bedding in to be laundered.

Posture and positioning while working

It is important that both you and your client are comfortable throughout the treatment.

All equipment and tools should be within easy reach so that you don't have to overstretch to reach them. The couch or chair should be at the correct height so that you don't have to reach too far up or down.

Your client should be placed in a comfortable position on the couch or chair. She should be able to remain relaxed during the treatment without having to twist or move so that you can reach her.

Celebrity and model make-up artists often apply their make-up using a special chair, called a director's chair. They need to be able to apply perfect make-up in an upright position.

Environmental conditions

Lighting

If the lighting is wrong, the effect of the make-up can be lost. If possible, apply make-up in the same light that the finished result is going to be shown.

For general day make-up, the best form of lighting is daylight. This allows the true colours to show and does not alter the natural colour that is applied. If daylight is not possible, the closest match is natural light bulbs arranged in an arch in front of the client. Professional make-up artists use this light to work in. The client should be positioned in front of the lighting arrangement so that no shadows are cast on her face that could affect the even application of the make-up.

Heating and ventilation

The make-up area should be warm enough so that the client is comfortable and the air conditioning should not make the environment feel stuffy. Clients don't need to undress to have make-up done so it is not necessary to have a very warm area as you would need to for facials.

> **» Get up and go!**
>
> Look at your make-up in different lights and see how the colours and effects change. Find out how make-up colours change in:
>
> - daylight
> - fluorescent light
> - spotlight
> - electric light bulbs.

Consult and prepare for make-up [1]

Before starting a make-up treatment, essential preparation is needed to make sure that you know what the client requires, are well prepared and have all the necessary equipment and products. Your equipment and work area must be clean, tidy and hygienic. The basic steps for getting ready for the client's make-up treatment are as follows:

1 Place all equipment and tools on a trolley that is easy to reach; it sometimes helps to lay them out in the order that you will use them so that this also helps to remind you of each step.

2 Set up your couch or chair with protective bedding.

3 Wash your hands.

4 Protect the client's clothing with a make-up cape or draped towel.

5 Protect the client's hair by placing a headband or sterile hair clip around the hairline.

6 Remove any large items of jewellery such as necklaces and earrings that you could accidentally catch.

7 Carry out a **consultation**.

8 If your client wears contact lenses, ask her if she would like to remove them.

9 Position the client in a **semi-reclining** position.

However, the first step before collecting your client is to set up your work area with all the materials that you will need. These are:

- brushes – a range of make-up brushes that you will need
- basics – the disposal products, laundry and workspace requirements
- products – all the creams and lotions needed for the make-up treatment.

Top tip ✓

You will need to wash your hands again before you start the make-up treatment on the client.

Brushes

A good set of brushes is very important, without these you will not be able to complete a professional make-up. Each stage of the make-up needs a different brush.

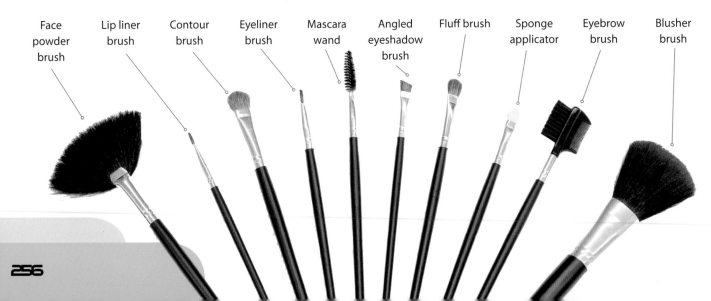

Face powder brush · Lip liner brush · Contour brush · Eyeliner brush · Mascara wand · Angled eyeshadow brush · Fluff brush · Sponge applicator · Eyebrow brush · Blusher brush

Item	Purpose
Face powder brush	The largest brush used to apply or blend face powder
Blusher brush	Used to apply blusher to the cheek area
Contour brush	Used for shading and highlighting the cheeks and face when you do corrective make-up
Eyebrow brush	A brush one side for brushing brows into shape and a comb the other side for separating lashes
Sponge applicator	Used for applying colour to the eyelids
Mascara wand	Used to apply mascara to the eyelashes
Angled eyeshadow brush	To apply colour or blend colour on the edges or sockets of the eyes
Fluff brush	Completes the blending as it is very soft and gets rid of any unblended edges
Eyeliner brush	To apply eyeliner or for blending eye pencil
Lip liner brush	To apply lipstick smoothly and perfectly

Basics

Item	Purpose
Cotton buds	For correcting any mistakes or make-up smudges
Eye pads (cotton wool circles or squares)	These rest on the eye while using a magnifying mirror for skin analysis
Cotton wool half moons	Cut from damp cotton wool pads, these are placed under the bottom lashes to protect the skin under the eyes from the make-up that is being cleansed off
Damp cotton wool squares	Used to cleanse the face
Tissues	Used for blotting excess toner, moisturiser and the first coat of lipstick
Dry cotton wool	Used to cover the tip of an orange stick which is then used to help remove make-up
Couch roll	Used to protect the client's clothing
Sponge wedges	Made of latex sponge and used to apply foundation to the skin
Make-up cape	Usually a velcro-fastened plastic cape that goes around the client's neck to protect her upper clothes from make-up spills
Headband or turban	To protect the client's hair from the products and to prevent her hair getting in the way of the treatment
Dishes	Small plastic or metal dishes are needed to hold cotton wool, tissues and the client's jewellery
Waste bin	A pedal bin with a lid is best for hygiene purposes, as you can open it without touching it with your hands
Spatula	A wide wooden stick that is used to scoop out cream or lotions from pots. Fingers should never be used as this is unhygienic and could spread germs
Orange sticks	Coat the ends with cotton wool as this softens the tips for safety when cleaning around the eyes
Palette	For decanting products on to and for mixing colours
Sharpener	To sharpen lip and eye pencils

Products

You might use any or all of the following make-up products:

- concealer - foundation - powder - blusher - eyeshadow - eyeliner
- eyebrow pencil - mascara - lip liner - lipstick - lip gloss.

Consult and prepare for make-up (2)

Client consultation

Before beginning any make-up treatment, you need to carry out a client **consultation**. This will involve the following.

- Questioning and recording information: this is when you ask the client questions about her skin and make-up routine and, importantly, why she would like to have her make-up done and what her wishes are. Asking for this information from your client will help you to understand what she needs from the make-up treatment and to find out about any colours or techniques that she does not like.

- Visual analysis: this is when you look at her face shape and skin type, as well as skin and hair colouring, to help you decide techniques and make-up types to use to complement the client's features. It is also important to look for any skin conditions and contra-indications.

- Manual analysis: this is when you feel the skin and decide whether it is dry or oily so that you can match the correct make-up to the skin type.

Remember that good communication skills are essential to conducting a professional consultation. Further information on communication methods can be found in Unit G3 Contribute to the development of effective working reationships.

Questioning and recording information

It is important to keep a record of a client's treatment, both during your consultation with the client and when you have completed the treatment.

The example of a consultation card on page 259 shows the information that you would typically record for a make-up treatment and why you need to record it.

> **Top tip** ✓
>
> If your client is under the age of 16, a parent or guardian must be present throughout the treatment. The parent or guardian must sign the consultation sheet to agree for the make-up treatment to go ahead – this is called giving consent.

> **》 Get up and go!**
>
> Look through celebrity magazines and choose a celebrity make-up that you like. Try to copy the look on a friend. Then take a photo of your friend and display it next to the magazine picture in your portfolio so that you can see if they look the same.

MAKE-UP CONSULTATION CARD

DATE 10/09/10   CLIENT'S NAME Mia Shaw

ADDRESS Flat 9, 12 Waterstone,   DATE OF BIRTH 24/03/89
Cambridge CB1 1NS

TELEPHONE NUMBER (H)   019924 555218   (W) 019924 213876

CONDITION OF SKIN ON INSPECTION
Mostly smooth and unlined but with dry patches

CONTRA-INDICATIONS/CONDITIONS
No contra-indications

EYE COLOURS AND PRODUCTS USED
Beige base, medium brown to add depth in the socket

Brown mascara

Brown eyeliner

CHEEK COLOURS AND PRODUCTS USED
Tawny blusher

FOUNDATION AND CONCEALER PRODUCTS AND COLOURS USED
Medium beige foundation and medium stick concealer

LIP COLOURS AND PRODUCTS USED
Nude lip liner and clear lip gloss

REASON FOR MAKE-UP   DAY ☑️   EVENING ☐   SPECIAL OCCASION ☐

HOMECARE ADVICE
Use a rich moisturising cream to help the dry patches

Cleanse, tone and moisturise twice daily

Use an eye make-up remover

PRODUCT SALES
Miss Gloss clear lip gloss

COMMENTS
Client really liked the natural day make-up and has booked to come
again as she has a birthday at the end of the month

CLIENT SIGNATURE

RECORD OF TREATMENTS
DATE	TREATMENT	THERAPIST
10/09/10	Day make-up	Pippa Lloyd

It is best to have a record of both the client's first name and surname. It is important to record the first name because there could be two clients with the same surname, which could cause confusion and lead to client records becoming mixed up.

Write the client's full address including the postcode.

Always write down a home number and a work or mobile number. One telephone number is not enough – if a client's appointment needs to be cancelled at short notice, you will not be able to contact her if she is at work and you only have her home telephone number.

Record any contra-indications or allergies in this section.

This is where you record the colours and types of make-up that you apply so that if the client wants the same make-up carried out another time you have the details. The client may also want to buy some of the products so it is important that you or someone else can refer to the record card to find out which products were used.

This is where you record any homecare advice that you give to the client.

This is where you record any products that you sell to the client so that if she returns to buy them again when she runs out the salon has details of what they were.

When you have finished the make-up treatment, this is where you record how you think it went and whether you and the client are happy with the results.

Dates, type of make-up and therapist's name should be kept as it may be useful in the future.

A typical consultation card for a make-up treatment

Consult and prepare for make-up [3]

Visual analysis

Once you have completed the paper-based part of the **consultation**, carried out a first visual study and questioned the client about contra-indications, you will need to thoroughly cleanse the client's skin and carry out a basic skin analysis. This includes finding out about:

- skin type
- skin condition
- contra-indications
- allergies.

This should be done in good light so that you are able to see well the skin's condition and texture.

Skin types and conditions

Skin types and characteristics such as colouring and condition vary between people. The type and characteristics depend on:

- age
- ethnic group
- gender.

When carrying out make-up treatments, you will need to consider all of these things as they will influence the colours, products and techniques that you will use on a client.

Age

Young skin is smooth and blemish-free whereas mature skin has lines and wrinkles, making make-up more difficult to apply.

Ethnic group

Different coloured skin means you will have to consider the colours that you use to complement it. For example, it would be unsuitable to apply a dark foundation colour to a light Caucasian skin.

- Caucasian skin is white and comes mostly from European origins.
- Oriental skin has a yellowish tone and is oily.
- Asian skin has a medium to dark tone with yellow base colour.
- African-Caribbean skin is dark and ranges in colour to almost black.

Gender

Female skin tends to be more sensitive and thinner than male skin, so more care will need to be taken when applying make-up.

Recognising skin types

Normal skin is rarely found in adults. It is usually found in children and young people. It:

- is smooth and clear with no blemishes
- is soft to touch
- has very tiny pores that are difficult to see.

This type of skin needs lots of gentle care to keep it normal.

Oily skin is caused when too much oil is produced in the skin. While we need oil to keep the skin smooth, when the skin produces too much it causes problems. Oily skin:

- has a shiny complexion with blackheads and blemishes
- has pores that are quite large
- means that the skin can be quite thick.

An oily skin can start or become worse as a teenager, when puberty hormones are most active.

Dry skin lacks oil because the oil glands in the skin do not produce enough. It:

- feels tight
- may flake and chap easily after washing, especially if soap is used
- soaks up creams and lotions easily
- can become lined and wrinkled early (especially around the eyes).

Dry skin must be moisturised well. Poor diet and not drinking enough water can cause dry skin or make it worse.

Combination skin is made up of two skin types. These types vary, but the most common is normal or dry skin on the cheek area, and an oily part on the nose and chin, and across the forehead (known as the **T-zone**). The oily T-zone shows up as a shiny nose, chin and forehead with blackheads.

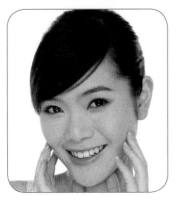
Normal skin

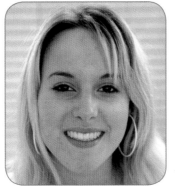
Oily skin

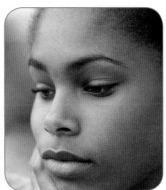
Dry skin

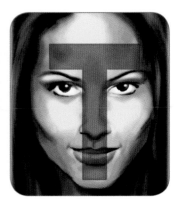
The T-zone

Matching make-up to a client's skin type

Make-up comes in many forms: pencil, liquid, powder, creams and lotions. It is best to match these where possible to a client's skin type. For example:

- a client with dry or mature skin should have cream-based make-up
- a client with oily skin should have a water-based foundation.

Consult and prepare for make-up (4)

Contra-indications

A contra-indication is a condition that makes or could make a client unsuitable for treatment. Not all contra-indications will prevent a make-up treatment being carried out. Some will just restrict treatment, in other words you can carry on with the make-up but will have to work around the area or go gently taking more care.

Here are some contra-indications that may restrict treatment and some advice for how to adapt your make-up treatment in line with these contra-indications.

- Healed eczema – this will present as very dry and parched skin and can quite often look very lined. Try to apply a very rich moisturiser before applying any make-up.
- **Psoriasis** – this is scaly flakes of skin, quite often red and inflamed. It is best to completely avoid these areas as the make-up will not go on smoothly and could make the condition worse.
- Redness – use a good concealer and covering foundation to balance the redness and steer away from using bright pinks and red, choosing instead neutrals, browns and greys to balance the redness.
- Bruising – use a good concealer to cover the bruising before applying further make-up. Apply it very gently as the bruise may be tender. If it is a very new bruise, you should work around it completely.

However, you must not treat a client who has contra-indications that could be made worse by treatment or could be spread to others.

The contra-indications that prevent you from carrying out your treatment include:

- blisters around the mouth and nose – this could be a cold sore
- bloodshot and watery eyes – this could be an eye infection
- extreme redness and/or inflammation – this could be a sign of an allergy, sunburn or an injury
- swelling or lumps – this could be bruising or something more serious
- dry, red and flaky skin, which could be eczema or **dermatitis**
- healing scars
- cuts
- skin irritation – it is recommended that you postpone the make-up treatment until the irritation goes as it could be a sign of an allergy.

The details about some of the contra-indications on pages 229–231 will help you to know what to look out for.

Dealing with contra-indications

If you notice anything unusual on your client's skin, you should ask your tutor or supervisor to check it for you before you start the treatment. Remember that you should never name a specific contra-indication when encouraging clients to seek medical advice and that you should make sure you do not cause the client to worry.

Contra-actions

Contra-actions are unwanted reactions that could occur during or after a make-up treatment. If these happen during the treatment, the treatment may need to be stopped mid-way through and steps taken to prevent it happening again in the future.

Allergies

Another very important reason why you may not be able to carry out a make-up treatment on your client is if they have an allergy to a product. As a therapist you need to be aware of this and take steps to keep your client safe and healthy.

Ingredients in cosmetics that could cause an allergic reaction include:

- skin care products – soaps and perfumes
- creams and lotions – **lanolin** (generally used in cheaper creams and lotions)
- lipsticks, face powders and blushers – dyes and colourings
- eyeshadows – powdered crushed glass (used to add shimmer)
- mascara and eyeliner – alcohol and fibres
- toning lotions – alcohol or citrus ingredients
- nail polish and removers – **acetone** and alcohol.

It is very difficult to pinpoint which product caused a reaction as you may have used several, but there are medical tests that can be done to find out the cause of the problem.

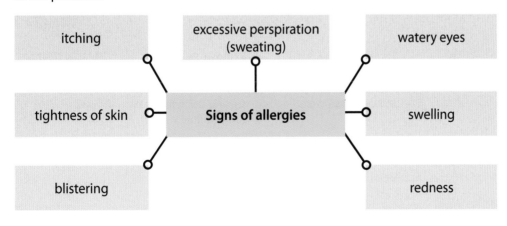

 Top tips

- You must always check for allergies before you apply any make-up because many cosmetic products contain **allergens**.

- If, after checking for allergies thoroughly beforehand, a client still reacts badly to a product by showing one of the signs, you will need to remove the product immediately and tell your supervisor, who will decide on the next steps that need to be taken. This will probably be to bathe the area with cool water and advise the client to see her GP.

Consult and prepare for make-up (5)

Preparing the skin

Before you can successfully apply any type of make-up, the skin must be very clean. Application of make-up on skin that has not been thoroughly cleansed and prepared could mean that the make-up will not last as long, will look uneven and will block the pores.

There are four steps to cleansing the skin thoroughly:

    1 eye make-up removal   **2** cleansing   **3** toning   **4** moisturising.

Eye make-up remover is a mild cleaning product that dissolves eye make-up so that it can be wiped off. The cleanser will remove old make-up, dirt, dead skin cells and oil from the skin – these also come in special **anti-bacterial** formulations for teenage or oily skin. The toner removes the cleanser, dissolves oil, cools and refreshes the skin while tightening it and closing pores. Finally, application of a moisturiser softens and protects the skin's surface while rehydrating it and providing a smooth base for make-up. You can find more information on all these products in Unit B2 Assist with facial skin care treatments.

Cleansing, toning and moisturising routine

This flow chart illustrates the steps that you should take in order to cleanse, tone and moisturise your client's face in preparation for her make-up treatment.

Start

Cleanse eyes
Place a half moon under the eye to stop the make-up staining the skin. Apply eye make-up remover to the lid using gentle circular movements. Stroke downwards to remove the make-up with a clean damp piece of cotton wool. Repeat until all the eye make-up is removed

Cleanse lips
Apply cleanser to the lips in small circles, using your little finger. Support one side of the mouth and sweep across with a clean piece of cotton wool from this side to the other and back again

First facial cleanse
Follow the routine illustrated on pages 238–242

Remove cleanser
With damp cotton wool squares using the same routine

Second cleanse
Follow the routine illustrated on pages 238–242 once more

Remove cleanser
With damp cotton wool squares

Apply toner
Put onto damp cotton wool and follow the cleansing routine to apply it

Blot toner
Using a split tissue, place it on the skin to soak up the excess toner

Repeat toning and blotting

Apply moisturiser
Apply using cleansing routine strokes

Wait for five minutes
Leave the skin to settle for five minutes and to give the moisturiser time to sink in. This is a good time to chat with your client about make-up colours

Finish

This diagram illustrates in detail the cleansing routine that you should follow.

Decant enough cleanser onto your hand to complete the first cleanse, spread it out between your hands and start the cleansing routine below.

1 Four stroking effleurage on the neck

2 Four stroking effleurage on the right cheek

3 Four stroking effleurage on the chin

4 Four stroking effleurage on the left cheek

5 Circles around the chin

6 Petrissage circles around the mouth and nose

7 Four stroking effleurage on the bridge of the nose

8 Four stroking effleurage on the forehead

9 Four eye circles (go in the direction of the eyebrow)

10 Finish with pressure on the temples before lifting hands off

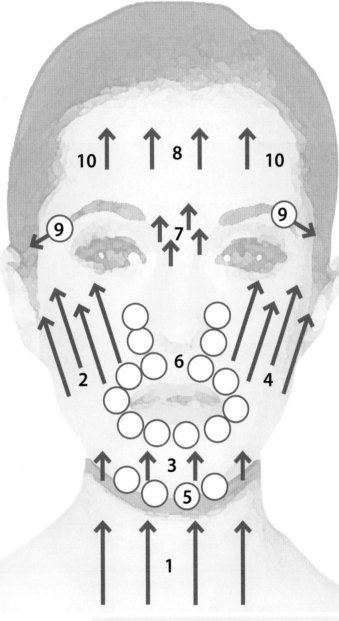

Cleansing routine

Move upwards, keeping in contact with the skin – do not lift your hands off

For step-by-step photos of how to cleanse, tone and moisturise a client's face, turn to pages 238–244 in Unit B2 Assist with facial skin care treatments.

>> **Get up and go!**

Find out where the words effleurage and petrissage come from.

? **Memory jogger**

1 What would happen if you applied make-up on uncleansed skin?

2 Give two disorders that may restrict a make-up treatment.

3 What is the difference between a contra-indication and a contra-action?

4 In what order should you carry out a make-up treatment?

A Cleanse, skin analysis, tone, moisturise, make-up

B Cleanse, tone, moisturise, make-up, skin analysis

C Skin analysis, cleanse, tone, make-up, moisturise

D Skin analysis, cleanse, make-up, moisturise, tone

Apply day make-up (1)

Although make-up may be used for a variety of effects such as theatre, television and photography, the techniques covered in this section are the first steps to developing skills as a make-up artist.

As with most things in life, for some people, make-up application comes naturally, whereas for others it can take a long time to perfect. At this stage, what is most important is to take care to not rush the application, and to think carefully about how to enhance the client's features and natural appearance. The steps and information outlined here will provide you with a solid base for developing more advanced technical skills in the future.

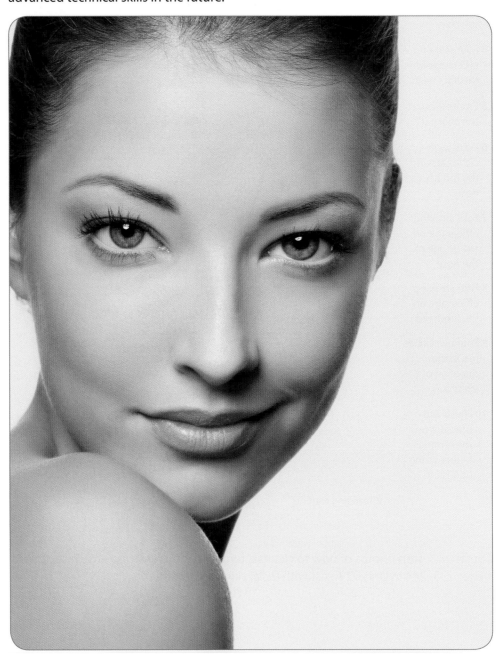

You need to think carefully about how to enhance features and create a natural appearance

Sequence of make-up application

To some extent, there are no set rules for the order in which you should apply make-up. It really depends on the products that are being used and the effect that is required. However, a common-sense approach to make-up application is important. The routine shown below would be a sensible way to go about it.

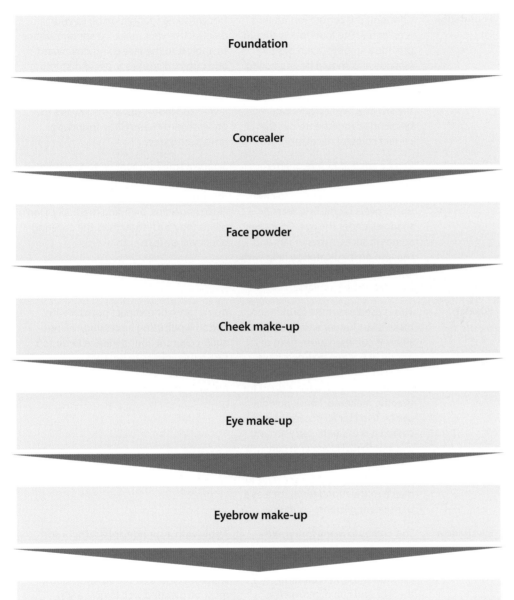

Foundation

Concealer

Face powder

Cheek make-up

Eye make-up

Eyebrow make-up

Lip make-up

A make-up routine

Some people prefer to apply eye make-up before cheek make-up and this is acceptable. However, if cream eye make-up or cream cheek make-up is used, this should be applied before face powder and not afterwards as in the routine above.

 Top tip

Never rush the first stages of foundation, concealer and powder application. It is these stages that prepare the skin for the colour – think of it as preparing your painting canvas.

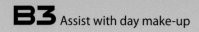

Apply day make-up (2)

Make-up products and application

Product	The basics	Application
Foundation	Choosing the correct foundation is essential. The foundation should provide a smooth, even base to work on and should be as close to the natural skin tone as possible. You should test the colour on the jaw line. Two colours can be blended together to get the correct colour if necessary.	Decant some foundation on to your palette. Use your make-up sponge wedge to apply it to the face using downward and outward strokes to avoid disturbing the tiny hairs on the face which could make the foundation go blotchy. Blend it well and fade it out at the jawline to prevent hard lines. A little foundation goes a long way.
Concealer	Can be applied before or after foundation depending on the type and how much you need to cover up. It covers blemishes, scars or shadows under the eye. Concealer comes in sticks, tubes or jars and can also be medicated to help with spots. It has a similar texture to foundation but is thicker.	Scrape a small amount on to a spatula, apply to skin using a brush, dotting in the required place. Then **stipple** using clean fingertips, blending gradually. Don't blend too much though as the covering effect will be lost.
Powder	This is used to set the foundation, make it last longer and to cut down shine. It comes in loose form or in a compact. Some powders have glitter or pearlised ingredients added to them, which are great for evening make-up. Loose powder can be used for all occasions, but compact is easier to carry around in a handbag. However, it can be unhygienic so should not be used by lots of people. Use a good match to the foundation, such as a translucent or transparent one.	Apply loose or compact powder with cotton wool, using a pressing/rolling action over the foundation. A large soft brush then needs to be used to brush off extra powder from the face so that it does not look too thick.
Eyeshadow	This comes in many forms and there are a whole range of colours and textures for use on the eyes. Eyeshadow brings colour to the face and can minimise less attractive facial features. Eye make-up can be used to correct features such as deep-set eyes. Effects can be soft or dramatic depending on the client's wishes or occasion, and it is not necessary to use the same colour as the eyes as they contain many different flecks of colour naturally.	Apply with a sponge applicator or soft brush. The lightest shade, the highlighter, is applied under the brow and the darker shadow colours on the lid. Eyeshadow must be blended well to give a soft appearance and professional finish.

Product	The basics	Application
Highlighter	This is usually powder-based and is a light colour such as white, beige or cream. It is used to highlight features.	Apply this to the arch of the eye with an eyeshadow applicator to open up the eyes. Also apply it to the cheeks using a blusher brush – it should be placed just above your blusher.
Eyeliner	Eyeliners go in and out of fashion regularly and are used to draw attention to the eyes. Eyeliner can be used to open, lengthen or add depth to the eyes depending on the type of application and colour. There are many types – liquid, cake, pencil or pen applicator.	Apply in a fine line as close to the roots of the lashes as possible. It can be applied to both the top and bottom lashes or either. To prevent hard lines, blend into eyeshadow by applying eyeshadow softly over the top. Use a damp cotton wool bud to clean up any smudges or mistakes.
Mascara	This makes the lashes look fuller and longer and comes in many colours and types; for example, some have fibres, some are waterproof. Some mascara can cause problems for clients with sensitive eyes or contact lens wearers, so always check for contra-indications and allergies before using.	Apply first downwards over the upper lashes, then ask client to look up slightly and stroke them upwards to coat underneath. Then coat the lower lashes. Keep a clean mascara comb so that you can separate any lashes that join together. Apply mascara in several thin coats rather than one thick coat and allow to dry between coats.
Blusher	This is used to give soft colour to the cheeks, create better shape and correct face shapes.	Apply powder blusher after the powder and cream blushers before powder. Apply with a brush to the cheek area, building up the colour slowly until you are happy with the result. Heavily applied blusher looks unnatural.
Lip liner	This is used to give a smooth outline to the lips and to correct the shape. Use a colour close to the natural lip colour if using a pale lipstick or clear lip gloss or, if using a brighter lipstick, use a liner the same colour.	Rest your little finger on the client's chin for support and gently outline the lips with the pencil. Do not ask the client to stretch her lips because when they relax and go back to normal the liner will be uneven and too dark.
Lipstick	This is the final touch to a make-up and brings the whole effect together. It adds colour and texture to the face as well as gloss and shine to the lips. Lipstick comes in many colours and textures, ranging from cream to pearlised and matt to glossy.	Scrape a little off the stick with a spatula and apply using a lip brush. Coat the outer part of the lips first and then fill in the centre. Blot with a tissue and then apply a second coat – this will give a better coverage and make the lipstick last longer.
Lip gloss	If applied to bare lips it gives a beautiful sheen or if used on top of lipstick it enhances the lipstick. It comes in many forms and colours.	Apply evenly with a lip brush, taking care not to overload the lips.

Apply day make-up (3)

Consequences of applying unsuitable make-up products

If make-up is applied incorrectly, the skin could suffer. Heavy-handed application of products could bruise the skin and it could also become sore and irritated. If a very sharp eye pencil was used around the eye, this could scratch the delicate skin around the eyes.

As well as poor application techniques, the wrong sort of make-up would be unsuitable. Deeply moisturising products on an oily skin would mean that the make-up would not last as it would come off easily. On the other hand, water-based products on dry flaky skin could make the make-up look patchy and uneven. Waterproof mascara that is difficult to remove or mascara with fibres in it could affect sensitive eyes. Using the wrong colours for skin type and characteristics will result in an unattractive make-up finish that is not right for the client.

Contra-actions

These are unwanted reactions to the make-up treatment. Certain products or techniques can cause problems, such as:

- redness
- rash
- soreness.

If your client shows any sign of these after you have applied a make-up product, you must remove it straight away and bathe the skin with cool water. The contra-action should calm down fairly quickly.

Other contra-actions that could happen are excessive perspiration, otherwise known as sweating, watery eyes and **erythema** (extreme redness).

How to treat contra-actions

Sweating: lower the temperature of the room, open a window, give the client a cool drink and stop the treatment until the sweating stops.

Watery eyes: give the client a tissue to dab at her eyes and wait until the watering stops before continuing with the eye make-up.

Erythema: this could be a sign of an allergy so stop using the make-up, remove it and bathe the skin with cool water.

> **? Memory jogger**
>
> 1 Give three examples of contra-actions.
> 2 Give three examples of contra-indications to make-up treatment.
> 3 Give three occasions when a client may want a make-up done.
> 4 Why should make-up be applied in a certain order?

Top tips ✓

- Always work with clean, sterilised equipment to prevent germs spreading.
- Work with care around the eyes as they are very delicate.

Step-by-step make-up

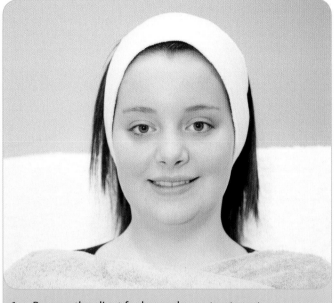

1 Prepare the client for her make-up treatment.

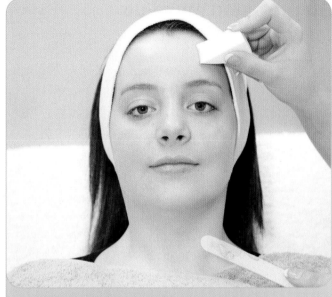

2 Apply foundation with a latex sponge wedge downwards and outwards.

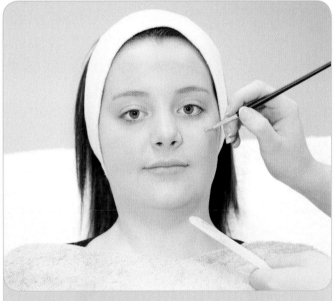

3 Apply concealer with a small brush and **stipple** it with a clean finger to blend.

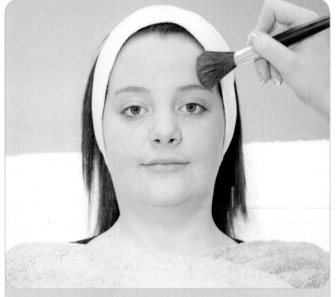

4 Set foundation and concealer by applying powder in a pressing and rolling action with a ball of cotton wool and dust the excess with a large soft powder brush.

Apply day make-up [4]

Step-by-step make-up

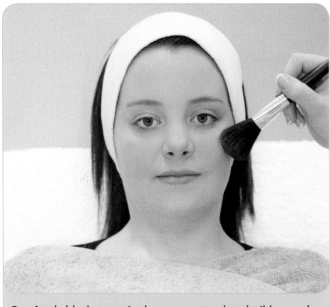

5 Apply blusher sparingly to prevent colour build up and a hard appearance.

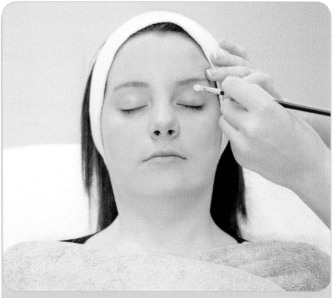

6 Use a sponge applicator to apply the highlighter under the brow bone.

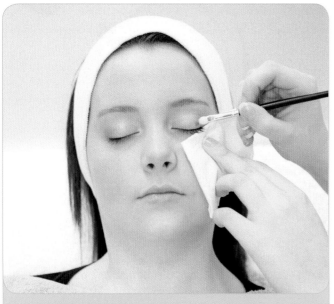

7 Add darker colour/s to the lid and blend afterwards with a soft eye brush.

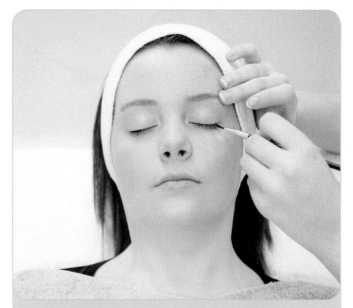

8 Apply eyeliner in a fine line as close to the lashes as possible. Blend with the eyeshadow to soften hard lines if desired. Then apply an eye pencil or shadow under the lashes to balance the eyes.

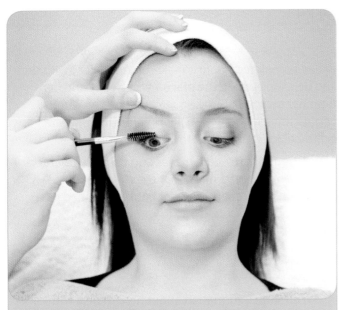

9 Apply mascara to the lashes using even, light strokes and comb through with a lash comb to separate the hairs.

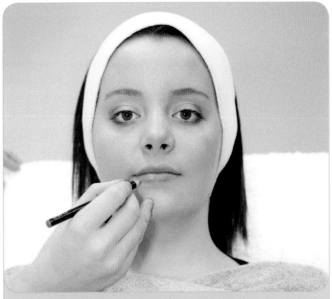

10 Balance your hand on the chin and gently apply the lip liner on the outside of the lips.

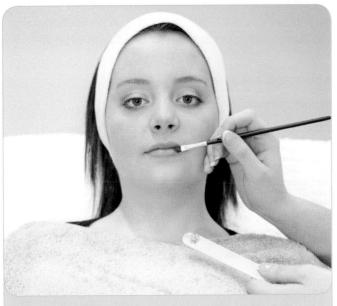

11 Complete the look by applying lipstick and lip gloss with a clean brush.

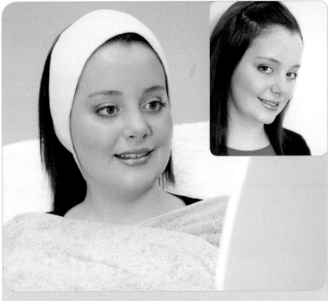

12 Show the client the mirror so that she can see the finished result.

Provide aftercare advice

It is important to remember that a treatment is not complete unless you have given your client some good advice for her to follow at home.

 Salon life

Emma was so pleased she had completed her first make-up on a client without the senior therapist helping her. She applied the make-up perfectly and her special sparkly mascara from her own make-up bag really set off the whole look. Emma's client went home thrilled with her make-up knowing that she would look great with her little black dress on for the party tonight.

However, as Emma's client was getting dressed her eyes and the skin around them started to itch. When she looked in the mirror her eyes had started to swell and were bloodshot. She looked dreadful and her flatmate gasped in horror. She rushed to the bathroom and rubbed off all her eye make-up, but the swelling did not go down – it just got worse.

Did Emma do anything wrong?

What should Emma's client do?

Had Emma's client been given enough information about how to deal with contra-actions?

Checking client satisfaction

A satisfied client will hopefully be a returning client, whether for make-up or something else, so it is important that you not only use good communication skills throughout the treatment but that you check that she is satisfied with what you have done.

During the application it is a good idea to check:

- that she is comfortable and warm
- that she is happy with the application so far – show her the progress in the mirror.

At the end of the treatment:

- show her the finished result in the mirror
- ask her if she is happy or if there is anything she would like slightly changed
- show her and explain the products that you used and where and how you used them
- offer to write the products down for her so that if she decides she would like to buy them she knows which ones to buy.

Homecare advice

Remember to give the following follow-up advice.

- Advise her not to touch her face too much as it will rub off the make-up.
- Advise her to make her make-up last longer by re-applying some powder and lipstick throughout the day.
- Advise her to remove her make-up very thoroughly before going to bed.
- Tell your client that if she has any contra-actions when she gets home or up to a couple of days afterwards, such as itchiness, irritation, redness or flaking, it may be that her skin has reacted to one of the make-up products. She will need to inform the salon and if the problem gets worse she must visit her GP.

Make-up removal techniques

Advise your client to gently use eye make-up remover, massaging it around the eye in circular movements and then using a cotton wool ball to remove the make-up and the eye make-up remover, taking care not to drag the eyes down.

For the face make-up, advise her on cleansing, toning and moisturising to ensure that all traces of make-up are removed and not left to block the pores.

Recording the treatment

All the techniques and colours used should be written on the client consultation card so that if the client returns for the same treatment you have a reference of the make-up used. She may also visit to buy some of the make-up products and if you have not written these down it is likely that you will have forgotten what you used.

 Get ahead

Design a make-up consultation card that can be given to a client at the end of her treatment. It should record the products used and how to use them.

≫ Get up and go!

Design your own make-up demonstration chart, with actual make-up colour smears, showing all of the colours that complement each other and that would blend well.

? Memory jogger

1 List three homecare pieces of advice that you could give to your client.
2 How can you check that the client is satisfied with the make-up treatment?
3 Describe how to remove eye make-up.

Getting ready for assessment

Evidence requirements

You will be observed by your assessor on at least three occasions, each involving a different client.

What you must cover during your practical assessments

Ranges

In your candidate handbook you will have a list of ranges that you must cover during your assessment. These ranges cover:

1 **consultation** techniques

2 skin types

3 client preparation

4 make-up products

5 advice.

It is good practice to cover as many ranges as possible during each assessment. This will prevent you having to take too many additional assessments because there are many ranges that you have not managed to cover.

Performance criteria

What you must demonstrate during a practical observation by your tutor:

- preparation for make-up
- a skin analysis
- good communication skills
- basic make-up application using:
  - foundation
  - concealers
  - powder
  - eye products
  - cheek products
  - lip products.

- checking the client is happy with the make-up treatment and finished effect
- giving aftercare advice to the client
- leaving the work area in a suitable condition.

Throughout your observations you will also need to make sure that you pay attention to health, safety and hygiene throughout, as well as presenting yourself well, so read through Unit G20 Make sure your own actions reduce risks to health and safety before any practical assessment just to refresh your memory.

Top tips ✓

- Make sure you are confident and have organised your work area, tools and equipment well.
- Prepare a checklist so that it is easy to check that you have everything to hand.
- Concentrate, don't let friends distract you.

Carrying out a practical treatment using unhygienic tools, or without carrying out a risk assessment of your work area to avoid accidents happening, will mean that you are not safe to do a treatment and therefore could mean that you do not pass your assessment.

What you must know

In order to pass this unit, you will need to gather evidence during the teaching and learning of this unit before your assessor observes your practical performance. You will gather this during classwork and further study and will probably file it in a portfolio of evidence. This evidence will also be signed off in your candidate handbook which you will be given by your assessor. This will be an official record to show that you have covered what you need to.

 Salon life

Jemima had an assessment today but had forgotten her make-up kit. Luckily she had her own make-up in her school bag so laid this out on her trolley when she was setting up for her client. Her friend Lucy lent Jemima some disposable eyeshadow applicators and lipliner brush, but did not have a disposable mascara brush.

Jemima started to apply a lovely day make-up using her own make-up and making do with the brushes she had in her own bag.

How could Jemima spread germs to her client by using her own make-up and brushes?

What infections could she pass on to her client by using her own make-up and mascara brush?

 Get up and go!

Cut out examples of make-up on celebrities from your magazines. Label the ones you like and say why, and the ones you don't like and say why.

Discuss with a partner how they could be improved.

UNIT N1

Assist with nail services

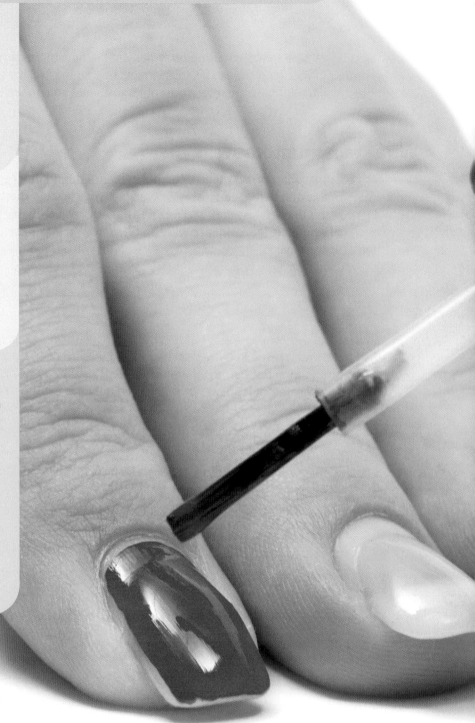

Well cared-for hands and nails are a great confidence booster. When a client looks down at her nails after a nail care treatment, she will notice a big improvement, even if she cares for them well herself. A professional nail care treatment is steps ahead of do-it-yourself treatments.

In this unit you will learn how to help with nail treatments and care for the nails on the hands and feet and surrounding skin. You will also learn about preparing for treatments and advising clients on aftercare.

In this unit you will learn how to:

- Maintain safe and effective methods of working when assisting with nail services
- Consult, plan and prepare for nail services with clients
- Carry out nail services
- Provide aftercare advice.

Here are some key terms you may meet in this unit:

Cuticle –
hardened skin at the base
of the fingernail

Manual labour –
work involving the hands

Scarf nail –
fine wisps of nail that
stick out after soaking

Methodical –
careful and organised, paying
attention to detail

Nail plate –
the hard, visible part
of the fingernail

Verruca –
a wart caused by a virus,
commonly found on the
feet and very infectious

Stress points –
the parts where the
nail is weakest

Athlete's foot –
a fungal infection commonly
found on the feet

Abrasive –
a rough and scratchy
substance that is used to
clean a smooth surface

Manicure station –
a trolley designed especially for
carrying out manicures

Bevelling –
a method of filing the nails
to reduce splitting

Hangnails –
dry strips of skin at the sides
of the nail that can become
very sore and inflamed if left
untreated or pulled off

Buffing –
polish and make shiny

Matrix –
the root of the nail

Pumice stone –
a special foot care tool
designed to remove hard skin

Maintain safe and effective methods of working when assisting with nail services [1]

Nail care treatments involve very close work and close attention to safe working practices is very important. However carefully you look after your nails at home, it is unlikely that you follow the high standards of hygiene expected of salon treatments. Some nail treatments use electrical equipment such as nail drills, files and dust extractors, which means that when you are assisting a therapist you need to be able to recognise safe working methods and follow instructions, even though you probably will not use electrical equipment yourself, as you may help to set them up.

The work area

Manicures

A manicure can be carried out in a variety of ways and some of these are better than others.

Some salons have an area especially set up for manicures, with good lighting and all equipment and products at hand. This is the best practice for manicure treatments.

In other salons a manicure is carried out in the reception area or as an extra part of a treatment. This is not best practice, and can be awkward for both the client and the therapist.

Here are the ways that a manicure can be carried out.

- Across a couch – with the client on one side and you on the other, and the products laid out next to you.

- At a **manicure station** – this is a trolley on wheels designed especially for carrying out manicures. It usually has drawers for storage and sometimes has a magnifying lamp. There should be room for the client to sit one side of the station and for the therapist to sit on the other side.

- The client sits in a couch or chair while the therapist sits on a manicure stool. The manicure stool has a cushioned seat, a swinging arm for resting and supporting the client's hands and arms and drawers underneath for the storage of products.

- The therapist sits to the side of the client while she is having her hair done. This is a very unsatisfactory way of carrying out a manicure. It is difficult for the therapist to carry out the manicure in comfort, which could affect the standard of the manicure.

- The therapist sits to the side of the treatment couch while the client has a facial. Again, this is not the best way to carry out a manicure. Either the client will have to stretch one of her arms across her body, or the therapist will have to swap sides to carry out the treatment on the second hand.

Pedicures

Setting up for a pedicure is more straightforward. The client usually sits on a professional chair that has a supportive back and the therapist sits in front.

Best practice is where the client's feet can rest on a special foot rest for pedicures. If a special foot rest is not available then the client can rest her feet on the therapist's lap, but this is less comfortable for both client and therapist.

Alternatively, well-equipped salons will have an electric-pedicure station, which is a large chair with built in foot bath and back massage facility for the client to enjoy during her pedicure.

As for any treatment, your work area must be organised with everything easy for you to reach. All items must be hygienic, with everything cleaned, disinfected and sterilised. Organise your products and tools in advance, and remember that it is helpful to arrange them in the order in which you will use them.

Top tip

When you set up, make sure that the tools and equipment are positioned so that you don't have to bend over to reach them. If you are right-handed, position the tools and equipment on the left. If you are left-handed, position them on the right. This helps to prevent you from knocking things over.

Get up and go!

Investigate a range of salon suppliers on the Internet to find out the different types of manicure and pedicure tools and equipment available for salons to buy. Print off some pictures of these for your portfolio.

Maintain safe and effective methods of working when assisting with nail services (2)

Sterilisation and cleaning of nail care tools and equipment

Maintaining standards of hygiene during nail treatments is extremely important. It is very easy to cause infection by using dirty tools and equipment. You must at all costs avoid allowing bacteria to enter the growing part of the nail through the **cuticle** or breaks in the skin.

Unit G20 Make sure your own actions reduce risks to health and safety explains in detail the difference between cleaning, disinfection and sterilisation, so refer back to this unit.

When setting up for nail treatments, you must follow these rules.

- All equipment must be cleaned with a detergent and then sterilised. The detergent removes the dirt and debris from their surfaces.

- Tools that need to be sterilised are things like cuticle knives, nippers and hard skin removers.

- All work surfaces must be disinfected using a spray or by wiping over with a disinfectant solution.

- Clean towels must be provided for each client and a biological detergent used so that they don't have to be washed at a very high temperature, which is not environmentally friendly.

- All creams, lotions and sprays used throughout the treatment should be decanted from pump-action bottles so that they are less likely to become contaminated with bacteria. If these are not available, a spatula must be used instead to remove the products from the container, bottle, tub or tube.

- Washing hands reduces the growth of germs and bacteria and also removes dust and dirt. Use a liquid soap in a pump-action bottle and paper towels as this is the most hygienic method. Always dry them thoroughly after washing as wet hands are not clean hands.

The table below shows how cross-infection could occur during a nail treatment.

Stage of the manicure or pedicure	Unhygienic practices that could lead to cross-infection	Potential result
Preparing to treat the client and/or during the whole of the treatment	Completing a treatment on one client and then carrying straight on to the next client without washing your hands, or handling money (money is covered in many germs) and then treating a client without washing your hands, or going to the toilet during the treatment and returning to the client without washing your hands.	Illness and skin infections
Soaking nails in warm soapy water	Using water that has previously been used on another client. The previous client may have had a **verruca**, or there may now be bits of skin floating in the water, either from the soles of the feet or the fingernails, which contain germs and dirt.	Veruccas and other bacterial, and fungal conditions such as **athlete's foot** and ringworm
Pushing back **cuticles**	Using cuticle tools that have not been sterilised and are covered in germs, which are then used on different clients.	Swollen and infected cuticles
Moisturising hands and feet	Using your fingers instead of a disposable spatula to scoop out the cream from the pot, meaning that after a few treatments the cream is full of germs from different clients.	Skin infections

Remember that the results of not being hygienic could be very damaging for both the salon and your career.

Maintaining hygiene throughout

You must remember that tools, equipment and you need to stay clean and hygienic throughout the treatment. The good hygiene and preparation procedures that you followed before starting are not enough, so you will need to make sure that:

- if you sneeze or cough you must cover your mouth and turn away from the client and then go and wash your hands
- if you blow your nose, wash your hands
- you don't put fingers in pots and containers of cream
- if you drop any nail tools or equipment, they must be cleaned and sterilised again
- you keep your work area tidy
- you throw away used tissues and cotton wool immediately in a nearby bin.

Leaving the work area clean and tidy

After you have finished the treatment and your client has left, it is essential that you clear away all of your tools and equipment and that you leave your work area clean and tidy. This will include:

- wiping over trolleys, couches, bins and stools with disinfectant
- cleaning your manicure tools and implements
- putting bedding in to be laundered
- tidying the work area for the next treatment or service.

» Get up and go!

Search the Internet for instructions and pictures showing how to wash your hands correctly. Choose the clearest picture and instructions, print it off and laminate it. Then put it by the sink in your classroom so that you have clear waterproof instructions for everyone to follow.

? Memory jogger

1 List three ways that you could cause cross-infection during your nail treatment.
2 What sort of detergent should be used to wash towels?
3 What are the three methods of reducing germs and bacteria?

Maintain safe and effective methods of working when assisting with nail services (3)

Checking that your equipment is in good working order

All equipment should be checked before starting the treatment so that it is safe to use, clean and works properly. You will need to check with your senior therapist or supervisor to make sure that everything is in good working order. Using poorly prepared equipment increases the risk of accidents in the workplace whereas dirty equipment could spread bacteria and cause infections.

Posture and positioning while working

As for any professional treatment, it is important that both you and your client are comfortable throughout the treatment.

During manicures and pedicures the therapist needs to bend over to carry out the service more so than other treatments, so it is especially important that you pay attention to your posture. It is important that you make sure that both you and your client are comfortable and that the height of the nail or pedicure station is easy to reach and does not make you lean over or bend too much. If your back is overstretched from reaching when carrying out the treatment, it will cause you back pain, neck ache and tiredness.

Therefore, once you have decided where you will be carrying out your nail service, you must make sure that:

- you and the client are not too cramped – there should be plenty of room for both of you to move your arms and legs freely
- the client is not positioned too far from you. You must be able to reach her hands and arms without having to lean over or stretch up.

Environmental conditions

Lighting

In order to see the **nail plate**, **cuticles** and polish during a manicure or pedicure, good overhead or natural lighting is essential. When carrying out the treatment, you should always check the following.

- Is the light bright enough?
- Does the light cast shadows?

This may be a particular problem if you are positioned in the corner of a room.

 Get up and go!

Set up for a nail treatment and then test different types of lighting on the area to see how much and how clearly you can see your tools, equipment and the nails of a friend.

Heating and ventilation

During nail treatments clients don't need to undress, but they will still take off their coat. For pedicures they will also either remove their trousers or skirt, or roll them up out of the way, so it is quite easy for them to get cold. Use a towel as a warm covering as well as for protection.

Although basic nail care treatments do not produce a lot of dust and vapour like artificial nail treatments, there is still the possibility that products such as nail varnish removers, acetone and varnishes could produce fumes that could overcome client and therapist. For this reason it is advisable to allow fresh air to circulate and during the winter, when perhaps this is not possible, a suitable method of artificial ventilation needs to be used.

As there is a possibility of fumes, you must remember to replace bottle tops immediately after use and use a pedal bin that closes properly for your waste.

 Top tip

Never leave cotton wool that is soaked in nail varnish remover on the work top. It will not only begin to dissolve a plastic nail station, it will also give off unwanted fumes.

? Memory jogger

1 What products could cause fumes during nail treatments?
2 How can you cut down fumes?
3 What is ventilation?
4 Why is it more likely for your back to ache during nail care treatments?

Consult, plan and prepare for nail services with clients [1]

The two keys to any successful nail treatment are good organisation and careful consideration of your client's needs. Clients will come to the salon for nail treatments for different reasons, so it is important for you to find out exactly what your client's wishes are. You will also need to look carefully at the nails and surrounding skin so that you can determine their condition and the nail shape, identify any problems and record details of the nail care routine that she follows at home. All this will help you to plan a suitable treatment for your client.

However, the first step before consulting with your client is to prepare your work area and set it up with all the materials that you will need. These are:

- basics – the disposable products, laundry and workspace requirements
- tech tools – the tools, such as scissors, that you will need
- products – all the creams and lotions needed for the treatment.

All of the basics, tech tools and products that you will need to assist with nail services are listed and explained on pages 287–289. Look back at pages 26–27 of Unit G20 Make sure your own actions reduce risks to health and safety to remind yourself of the correct procedures for cleaning, disinfecting and sterilising tools and work surfaces.

To make sure that you keep the tools and equipment needed for nail services in good working order, make sure that you:

- clean and sterilise them after every client
- only use tools made for professional nail services
- oil the hinges and screws regularly to stop them becoming stiff.

 Top tip

It helps to have a checklist of the tech tools, products and nail basics on a record card that you can keep nearby for reference. Cover the list with a plastic cover so that it does not get marked, or have it laminated so that you can wipe it clean.

 Get ahead

Design and carry out a survey to find out how often clients have their nails done professionally and the sorts of nail services they have. Discuss the findings with your friends and tutor.

Basics

Item	Purpose
Cotton wool	To remove nail varnish, the cotton wool is rolled into small balls and each ball is soaked with nail varnish remover. A clean piece of cotton wool is used for each nail. Cotton wool is also used to cover the tip of an orange stick, for **cuticle** work, the application of cream and nail cleaning.
Tissues	Tissues are used for various things during a manicure, such as wiping products from the nail. Tissues are normally made up of two very thin layers (two-ply). In a salon, tissues are split (one-ply) as this makes them more economical to use.
Towels	A towel is used to dry the hands and fingers or feet and toes of the client after they have been soaked in water during a manicure or pedicure. Towels are also used to protect a client's clothing if she is not wearing a gown.
Gown	The client may wear a gown to protect her clothing from spills or splashes of a product, or you may place a protective towel over her clothing instead.
Dishes	Small plastic or metal dishes are needed to hold cotton wool and tissues, as well as the client's jewellery. Any jewellery left on during a manicure will get in the way of the treatment and become coated in hand cream.
Waste bin or container	A pedal bin with a lid is best for hygiene purposes, as you can open it without touching it with your hands. However, if you are doing a manicure or pedicure in a corner of a room or an area without a pedal bin, then you can use a waste paper bin lined with a disposable bag. After the treatment, make sure that the bin is emptied, and the bag is sealed and placed in a waste bin with a lid. If a bowl or container other than a bin is used for waste, make sure that you have lined it with couch roll first. This will allow you to scoop the waste up easily after the treatment. Remember to wash and disinfect the bowl afterwards.
Sterilising jar	This should be filled with antiseptic or disinfectant solution, so that small metal tools that have been previously sterilised can be placed in it during the treatment. The solution will help to keep germ levels down, but it will not destroy germs completely. The solution should be changed after every client.
Manicure cushion	These provide extra comfort during the manicure. They allow the client to rest her hands and also give support to the wrist. Cushions are not usually used for pedicures as the foot is supported on a foot stool or pedicure station. Manicure cushions usually have a removable washable cover made from towelling. However, if the cushion does not have a cover, then a protective towel should be placed on top.
Manicure or pedicure bowl	The manicure bowl is a specially shaped gripper bowl, which has a small hole in it for the thumb and a larger hole for the rest of the fingers. It is filled with warm soapy water in which to soak the client's hands during the manicure. It has a removable lid so that it can be cleaned thoroughly inside after each treatment. For the pedicure a shaped foot bowl is sometimes used, or at other times a foot spa or built-in foot bath.

Consult, plan and prepare for nail services with clients (2)

Tech tools

When setting up for a nail service, you need to prepare all the tools you will need.

Item	Purpose
Spatula	A spatula is used for scooping out products hygienically.
Emery board	This is a thin card file with an **abrasive** covering on each side. It is used for filing and shaping the nails. The fine side is used for fingernails and the coarse side for male manicures and toenails, as they tend to be thicker than fingernails. Emery boards come in different sizes and widths, and some have funky designs on them. They should be disposed of after use, for hygiene purposes.
Orange sticks	These are made of orange wood, which is slightly bendy. One end is pointed and the other end is shaped like a hoof. Both ends of the orange stick are coated in cotton wool for hygiene purposes, as the cotton wool can be removed and thrown away after use. The cotton wool also softens the tip, which prevents the **cuticles** and skin becoming sore during treatment. The pointed end is used for cleaning under the free edge of the nail and the hoof end is used for cuticle work.
Rubber hoof stick	In addition to the orange stick, this tool can also be used to push back the cuticles safely. At the end of the wooden stick is a hoof-shaped rubber piece. However, once it has been sterilised a few times, the rubber tends to fall apart, so the hoof stick needs to be replaced regularly.
Nail brush	This can be used during the nail soaking to gently rub away staining around the fingers or toes or on the nails. It is also used to take off cuticle remover. However, it is not a very hygienic tool as it is extremely difficult to sterilise completely and can harbour germs between the bristles.
Nail buffer	This is made of chamois leather and is used with a buffing paste to shine the **nail plate**. The action of the **buffing** also improves the blood flow to the nails, which encourages nail growth.
Nail scissors	These are curved scissors that can be used to cut long nails before filing if it would take too long to use an emery board.
Cuticle knife	This blunt, straight-edged tool is used to gently free any cuticle that has stuck to the nail plate. This is done by applying light pressure and making small circular movements at the base of the nail. When using this tool, you should be careful not to use a digging and pushing-back action, as this will only damage the **matrix** and make the cuticles sore. You should know about the instrument, but you will not be using it at Level 1.
Cuticle nippers	These cutting tools do not cut the main part of the cuticle, as the name suggests. Instead, they are used gently to cut away extra skin that has grown down the nail from dry, uncared-for cuticles. They are used only after the cuticle has been softened and loosened with cuticle remover and a hoof stick or cuticle knife. You should know about the instrument, but you will not be using it at Level 1.

Products

When setting up for a nail service, you need to make sure you have all the products you will need.

Product	Purpose
Nail varnish	This is used to colour or give shine to the nails at the end of the nail care treatment. They come in many colours, effects and types.
Nail varnish remover	This dissolves nail varnish so that it can be wiped off the **nail plate** easily with a piece of cotton wool. Nail varnish remover has a drying effect on the nail so it usually contains a small amount of oil to moisturise it.
Cuticle cream	This is a thick moisturising cream that is used to soften and nourish the **cuticle** so that the cuticle can be pushed back more easily during a nail care treatment without the skin splitting or pulling.
Cuticle remover	This is a milky-coloured liquid that contains an active ingredient to dissolve skin cells. It is used to loosen any cuticle that sticks to and grows along the nail plate. It also acts as a nail shampoo because it contains an active ingredient to bleach out stains. The senior therapist will demonstrate and carry out this part of the nail treatment.
Buffing paste	**Buffing** paste contains an **abrasive** ingredient that is used to smooth out fine ridges on the surface of the nail. It also helps to remove surface stains on the nail plate. Buffing paste leaves the nails with a shiny surface and can be used instead of nail varnish.
Moisturiser or massage cream	This is a rich cream that is massaged into the hands and arms or feet and lower legs at the end of the manicure or pedicure and before the nail varnish is applied.
Nail varnish dryer	A nail varnish dryer does not dry the nails completely, but it helps the varnish to harden more quickly. It comes in the form of a spray or paint-on-product (similar to clear nail varnish) and can be oil- or alcohol-based.

>> Get up and go!

How many nail basics, lotions and creams, and tech tools can you remember? In pairs, look at each list for one minute. Then test each other's memory.

? Memory jogger

1 How should you cut a nail to prevent damage to the layers?
2 Name two tools that you will not use for Level 1.
3 The skin around the nails is removed with:
   A Cuticle remover
   B Cuticle massage cream
   C Acetone
   D Buffing paste
4 Give two uses of an orange stick in nail care treatments.
5 What is the purpose of cuticle moisturising cream?

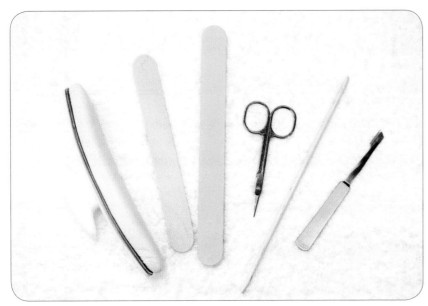

A selection of nail tools

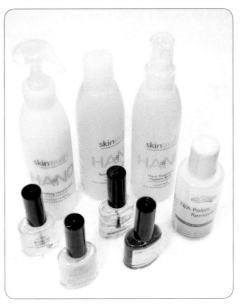

A range of hand and nail treatments

Consult, plan and prepare for nail services with clients (3)

Client consultation

A client consultation must be carried out before a manicure or a pedicure, just as for any other salon treatment. There are many reasons why a client may book a nail care treatment and it is not only clients with good nails and surrounding skin who come to the salon for this treatment. Consulting with your client will allow you to find out what she would like and to decide, based on the condition of the client's nails and skin, how to go about your treatment.

The consultation involves the following three stages:

- questioning and recording information
- visual analysis
- manual analysis.

Questioning

Here are some of the reasons why clients come to a beauty salon for nail treatments. Remember that men may also come to the salon for a male manicure or pedicure.

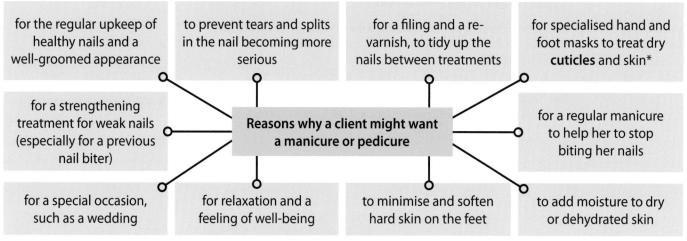

for the regular upkeep of healthy nails and a well-groomed appearance	to prevent tears and splits in the nail becoming more serious
for a strengthening treatment for weak nails (especially for a previous nail biter)	
for a special occasion, such as a wedding	for relaxation and a feeling of well-being

Reasons why a client might want a manicure or pedicure

for a filing and a re-varnish, to tidy up the nails between treatments

for specialised hand and foot masks to treat dry **cuticles** and skin*

for a regular manicure to help her to stop biting her nails

to minimise and soften hard skin on the feet

to add moisture to dry or dehydrated skin

* These are not covered in Level 1

Reasons for manicures and pedicures

You need to ask to ask this information of your client to help you understand what she needs. For hand treatments, it is also important to ask about the client's lifestyle and job. This will help you to understand how much the client uses her hands and will tell you whether she is able to grow her nails long or needs to keep them short.

Visual analysis

This is when you look at the client's hands or feet, nails, skin colour and texture. It involves a thorough look at the nails and surrounding skin to find out information such as condition and strength of the nails and the condition of the skin and cuticles, as well as looking for anything that looks like a contra-indication.

Manual analysis

This will be carried out after completion of the paper-based part of the consultation, in which you take down client details and carry out a first visual study. You will need to clean the client's hands or feet and nails as well as your own hands by wiping over with a skin and nail cleaner or a hygienic spray. When you have done this you will be able to touch the client's hands or feet and nails in order to check them for the condition of nails, **cuticles** and skin, and any contra-indications and conditions.

This should be done in good light so that you are able to see well the nail and skin condition and texture. You must also write down what you see and feel on the client's record card.

Assessing the condition of a client's hands: a checklist

1 Examine the front and the backs of the hands.
2 Look at the colour and texture of the skin – is it tanned or light? Is the skin thin or thickened?
3 Are the hands soft and smooth or are they rough and chapped?
4 Does the skin show any signs of infection such as swelling, pus or lifting of the **nail plate**?
5 Are there cracks and breaks in the skin or redness around the cuticles?
6 Look at the skin between the fingers – are there any signs of dryness?

Assessing the condition of a client's feet: a checklist

1 Examine the top and underneath of the feet, looking carefully at the condition of the skin on the heels.
2 Look at the colour and texture of the skin – is it tanned or light? Is the skin thin or thickened?
3 Are the feet soft and smooth or are they rough and chapped?
4 Does the skin show any signs of infection such as swelling, pus or lifting of the nail plate?
5 Are there cracks and breaks in the skin or redness around the cuticles?
6 Look at the skin between the toes – are there any signs of dryness or moisture which could be an indication of athlete's foot, a fungal infection?

Assessing the condition of a client's nails: a checklist

1 What shape are the nails?
2 What length are the nails? Are they long or short? Have they been picked or bitten?
3 Are the nails healthy – strong, pink, shiny and flexible? Are they unhealthy – yellow, brittle, weak and thin?
4 Do the nails show any signs of nail diseases or disorders?
5 Is there any lifting of the nails, which could suggest nail disease or fungal infection?
6 Are the cuticles hard and overgrown, red and inflamed or smooth and even?
7 Have the cuticles grown along the nail plate?
8 Are there any **hangnails**?

Consult, plan and prepare for nail services with clients (4)

Contra-indications

A contra-indication is a condition that makes or could make a client unsuitable for a treatment. It could be unsafe to treat a client with a contra-indication. At Level 1 you are not responsible for deciding whether or not a client has a contra-indication, but you must be aware of them and be able to recognise the signs so that you can tell a senior therapist if you notice anything unusual.

Whatever level of experience therapists have, they are not qualified to diagnose medical conditions. You may have an idea of what medical condition a client may have, but the appropriate action is to refer them to their GP. You must also make sure that you do not cause the client alarm or embarrassment by talking loudly about a contra-indication so that other people may hear.

Look out for the following contra-indications. You should also look out for **athlete's foot** (which is a type of ringworm) and **verrucas** when you inspect your client's feet before a pedicure.

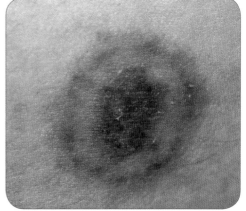

Warts

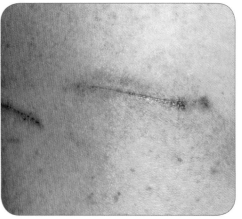

Ringworm

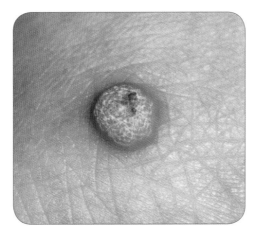

Scabies

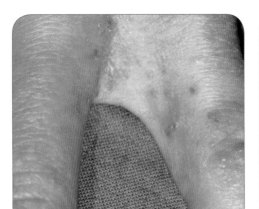

Cuts and abrasions

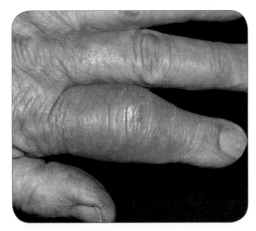

Swelling and inflammation

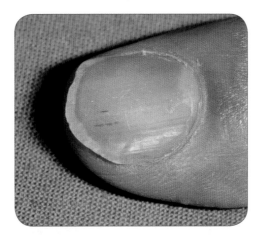

Damaged nails

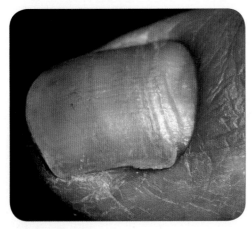

Discoloured nails

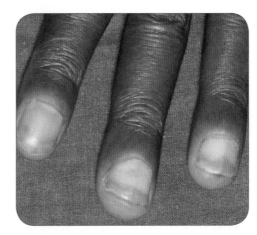

Overgrown cuticles

 Top tip

Always ask a senior member of staff to double check that you have not overlooked any infection or problem.

Get up and go!

Find as many photos of nail contra-indications as you can on the Internet. Google Images is a good place to start.

? Memory jogger

1 What is a contra-indication?

2 Why must you not diagnose a condition?

3 Name two contra-indications you may find on the feet.

4 Name two contra-indications you may find on the hands and nails.

Consult, plan and prepare for nail services with clients (5)

Recording information

Once you have completed a full consultation and before you start any treatment, you will need to record the answers and information on the client's record card. You will need to record what the client tells you about her wishes and nail care routine, and also your own observations from the visual and manual analyses. When you have completed the treatment, you will need to complete the card.

MANICURE/PEDICURE CONSULTATION CARD

Date 16/11/10   Name Jon Bomero

Address Westbrook, St Giles Road,   Date of birth 23/06/89
Tonmouth GR7 4EL

Telephone Number (H) (01121) 556600   (W) (01121) 818120

Condition of Hands/Feet/Nails on Inspection

Hands – dry and chapped

Nails – cuticles dry and overgrown. Nails thick and stong

Contra-Indications/Conditions

None

Products Used

Simply Men manicure range

Product Sales

Homecare Advice

Carry out a salt and oil rub to help remove dry skin but avoid any chapped areas. Use moisturiser daily.

Comments

Removed excess cuticles, buffed nails.

Advised client to return monthly.

Client Signature

[signature]

Record Of Treatments

Date	Treatment	Therapist
13/01/10	Manicure	S Jones
16/11/10	Manicure	Nadia Hoffmann

A typical consultation card for a manicure or pedicure treatment

---

You will need to record the following.

- Client's contact details – name, address and telephone numbers. Make sure that you write down both the client's first name and surname, the postcode and a work or mobile telephone number as well as a home number. This will help to avoid confusion if you have more than one client with that surname, and will mean that you will be able to get hold of the client no matter where he or she is if you need to contact them at short notice to let them know about a change in appointment time.

- The client's wishes and information about their job and lifestyle.

- The condition of nails and hands or feet when inspected.

- Any allergies.

- Any contra-indications.

- The products used during the treatment:
  - write down any extra products, apart from the products you would always use in a manicure or pedicure, that you use on the client, such as nail strengtheners and ridge fillers
  - you should also list the varnish colour you use in case the client asks for the same colour the next time she comes to the salon.

- Advice given to the client:
  - what advice did you give your client on how they could improve the condition of their hands and nails?
  - when did you advise her to return for another salon treatment?
- Any products you sell to the client.
- Any other comments:
  - what were the results of the manicure?
  - have you any advice to other therapists? Include whatever you think may be useful to you or another therapist in the future.
- Record of treatments:
  - the date
  - the type of manicure
  - the therapist's name
  - any extra notes that could be useful for the future.

Client's consent

You must always get your client to sign the consultation to agree for the nail treatment to go ahead – this is called giving consent.

Treating a minor

If your client is under the age of 16 a parent or guardian must be present throughout the treatment and they (the parent or guardian) must sign the consultation card to give consent for the treatment to take place.

Preparing the client

Once your work area is set up, you can collect your client and ask her to sit down so that you can prepare her. The first thing you should do is wash your hands. Then place a towel over any clothing that could become marked by water or the nail care products.

Remove any items of jewellery, dress rings, bracelets, ankle bracelets and toe rings. Once you have carried out the consultation, you can help your client into the manicure or pedicure chair, making sure her position is comfortable for both of you.

Before you begin the nail manicure treatment: a checklist

1 Make a quick check of your workplace preparation.
2 Wash your hands.
3 Remove both your own and your client's watch and jewellery.
4 Protect the client's clothing.
5 Carry out a consultation.
6 Assess the condition of your client's hands and nails.
7 Check for contra-indications.

 Get up and go!

Take a photo of your fully prepared work area. Include it in your portfolio to show a good set up.

? Memory jogger

1 Why is it important to record the answers your client gives you during consultation?
2 List four things that should be recorded on a client record card.
3 What age is a minor?

Carry out nail services (1)

Before you carry out any nail treatment, it is very important for you to understand the structure, parts and functions of the nail. Pages 210–211 of the Anatomy and physiology section of this book contain all the information you need to know.

Nail shapes

Nail shapes vary from one client to another. The natural nail shape usually mirrors the line of the **cuticle** (see the diagrams of the different nail shapes).

When shaping nails, you need to think about the following:

- the shape of the existing nail – you cannot change the natural shape of the nail, you can only improve it
- the client's lifestyle and job – for example, is she or he sporty or do they do manual work, in which case are long fingernails really practical? In the case of toenails, if the client does a lot of running, they should be short so that they don't become squashed up in trainers which could result in bruised nails
- what the client wants – clients usually have a good idea of how they want their nails to look and what needs doing. Alternatively, they may be going somewhere special and want them painted a certain colour to match an outfit
- the shape of the cuticles – when shaping the nails, follow the cuticle line for a natural look, unless the client wishes to follow the current fashion in nail shapes.

Fingernail shapes

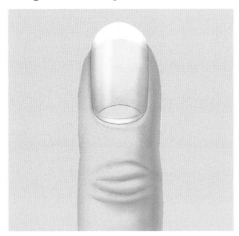

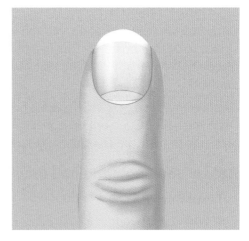

Oval

This all-purpose nail shape flatters and softens the appearance of the hands. It makes the fingers look longer. It is also quite hardwearing against breakage because of its smooth edges and flexible shape.

Round

This is also a very practical nail shape. It is hardwearing, strong and neat. However, it is not very flattering as it does not help to make the fingers look longer.

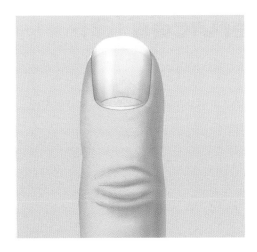

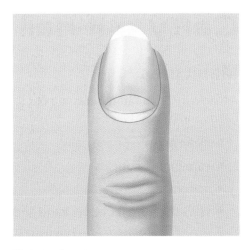

Square

This is a very good shape if the nails are short and the fingers quite long. This shape is also less likely to break because the nail wall provides good support for the sides of the nails. It is therefore ideal for people who do **manual labour**, such as typists, medical staff and cleaners. However, it is not a good shape on short fingers, as it can make them appear even shorter.

Pointed

Some clients prefer this nail shape as they believe it makes their nails look longer. However, it is best to advise against this shape as the nails are filed to a point from the corners to the tip. The corners where the free edge starts are the **stress points** of the nails – the nails have no support from the nail wall so can easily weaken and split.

Toenail shapes

These tend to be naturally square or rounded. When shaping them during a pedicure, they must be filed or cut straight across making sure you don't shape them into the corners as this can cause ingrown toenails.

 Get up and go!

Look at the different fingernail shapes on your fellow students. Which are the most common?

? **Memory jogger**

1 List three fingernail shapes.

2 How should you shape a toenail?

3 How will you decide what shape to do the fingernails?

Carry out nail services (2)

Manicures

A manicure is a treatment carried out to improve and beautify the condition of the hands and nails. It takes about 30–45 minutes to complete and its aims are to:

- clean and shape the nails
- care for the **cuticles**
- soften dry skin on the hands
- relax the muscles in the hand and arm
- give a healthy shine to the nails.

A manicure includes the following:

- a hand and nail inspection – to check the condition of the hands and for any problem areas
- filing and **bevelling** – to neaten the nails and remove splits and catches
- soaking – to soften the skin for cuticle work
- cuticle work – to push back and neaten the cuticles
- massage – to moisturise the skin, improve blood flow and relax the client
- **buffing** – to smooth ridges, give a healthy shine and improve the blood flow
- painting – to beautify the nails by adding colour and shine.

After a manicure, the nails should look naturally polished or perfectly painted. The skin on the hands and around the cuticles should be soft and smooth.

Step-by-step manicure

This diagram illustrates the stages involved in a manicure.

Top tips ✓

- Explain to your client what you are doing as you go along and why, because it is important to keep the client informed.
- Chat to the client about her wishes for today's treatment. Remember that these can change from one week to the next, so remember to check each time.

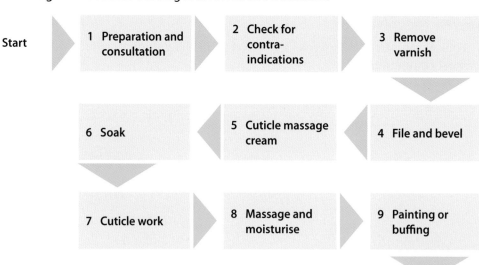

Summary of steps in a manicure

Removing nail varnish

When you have carried out your consultation and prepared your client for her manicure, your first step is to clean the client's nails and remove any varnish she might have on.

 Top tips

- A fresh piece of cotton wool should be used for each nail, because once there is a build-up of dissolved varnish on the cotton wool ball, it is not as good at removing varnish.
- Nail varnish tends to stain around the cuticle and nail fold, so use a covered orange stick dipped in nail varnish remover to remove the varnish from these areas.

Filing and bevelling

Do not saw in both directions, as this will cause the nail to split. Use the file at a 45° angle to the nail and file from one side of the nail to the centre, then file from the other side to the centre.

Top tip

If the nails are very long and need cutting, this is best done after they have been softened by soaking in water. Cutting hard, dry nails will cause the nail layers to separate and the nails to split.

45° angle

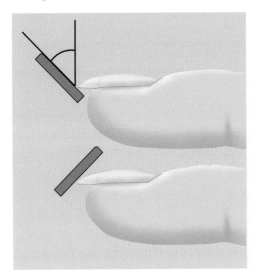

File the nail at a 45° angle

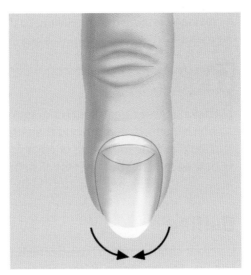

Side-to-centre action

Cuticle work

Cuticle cream both softens the **cuticles** so that they are easier to push back and moisturises dry skin and nails. It also acts as a nail shampoo and will help get rid of staining or stubborn dirt. Place any loose bits of cuticle or dirt on a tissue and throw it away afterwards.

Cuticle remover must be wiped off thoroughly, otherwise it may carry on working and could cause soreness.

Top tip

Scarf nail is the name for fine wisps of nail that stick out after soaking. They are very flimsy and thin, like a scarf.

Carry out nail services (3)

Massage and moisturise

Moisturising softens and smoothes the skin and is a perfect finish to a manicure. The moisturiser or massage cream is applied and rubbed into the skin using rubbing and kneading movements (see page 309).

A simple massage routine is to start with lighter strokes that become deeper. Begin with the arm up to the elbow, then move down to the hands and the fingers. The hand and arm massage routine should take about five to ten minutes to complete on both hands.

After you have carried out a massage using a rich moisturising or massage cream there may still be some cream on the nail. If it remains on the nail, the nail varnish will not go on smoothly and will not dry properly. If you do manage to paint nail varnish on the nails, the varnish will soon peel off once you have finished. It is therefore very important that you degrease the nails thoroughly with nail varnish remover following the massage.

 Top tip

For Level 1, it is not necessary for you to follow a set massage routine using all the movements. However, it is important that you carry out some sort of massage routine that is relaxing to the client.

 Get ahead

Plan a six-week treatment programme for one of your friends, family or clients which is aimed at improving the skin and nails of their hands or feet. Your plan should include full details of what you will do during each of the six weeks and how each of the treatments will help them.

Buffing

If a client chooses not to have her nails painted, offer to buff them for her. This will improve the circulation in her nails and polish them, leaving a healthy, natural shine.

 Top tip

Do not rub while **buffing** as this will create heat, which can be painful as well as damaging to the layers of the nail. Do about four to six strokes on each nail in a downward direction. Do not be tempted to do any more strokes.

Painting

Top tip

If the client wants a varnish, now is the time to ask her to put all her jewellery back on, to put on her jacket or coat, and to get her car keys out of her handbag. You should also politely ask if she would like to pay for the manicure before you paint her nails, explaining about the drying time of varnishes.

Nail varnish should be painted on in a **methodical** way. Here is a guide to show you how best to do this.

Painting your client's nails

1 Make sure that your client's nails are very clean – there should be no dirt or grease on them.

2 Prepare a cotton wool-coated orange stick by soaking it in nail vanish remover. This is in case you make a mistake while painting or to clean off any varnish around the **cuticle**. It is better to remove the nail varnish straight away, because wet nail varnish is easier to remove than dry nail varnish.

3 Paint the nails. While painting, support the client's hand while holding the nail varnish bottle and complete the strokes with your other hand.

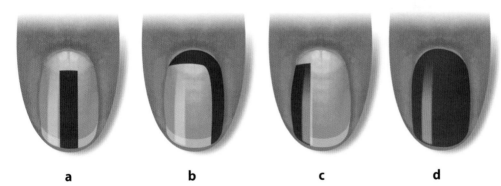

Painting the nails

a   **b**   **c**   **d**

When painting the nails:

a begin with one central application

b then apply the varnish to the right

c then apply the varnish to the left

d go over the whole nail to smooth the varnish.

Carry out nail services (4)

Painting tips

Do:

- make sure that you have enough varnish on the brush to do the whole nail
- paint thinly
- use only a few strokes
- leave a small gap at the base of the nail before the **cuticle**
- hold the bottle while you paint.

Don't:

- overload the brush with paint, as it will drip down and flood the nail with too much varnish
- paint thickly, as it will take too long to dry
- use too many brush strokes, as the finish will be lumpy and uneven
- paint right up to the cuticle, as the varnish will seep into the skin and look messy
- dip the brush in a bottle that is not held, as it could fall over and spill varnish.

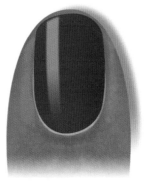

While painting, leave a small gap at the base of the nail before the cuticle

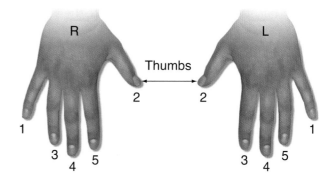

To prevent smudging, follow the finger rotation method

Start	1 Replace client's jewellery and take payment	2 Choose colour	3 Degrease nails
6 If cream varnish, apply top coat	5 Apply two coats of varnish		4 Apply base coat
7 Apply nail dry	Finish		

Summary of steps involved in painting nails

Polish profile

Base coats

These can be clear or pale coloured. They are applied to the **nail plate** before varnish to:

- smooth the nail
- cut down on staining from bright coloured varnishes
- help prevent early chipping or the colour wearing off.

Top coats

These are usually clear and are used to:

- give a high shine to the coloured nails
- help to make the varnish last longer.

Some top coats also have an added ingredient which helps to speed up the drying time.

Ridge-filling base coats

These are usually pale in colour and thicker than normal base coats. If a client has a very uneven nail plate with ridges or dips, the ridge filler will help to smooth the surface of the nail.

Nail hardeners

These are clear varnishes but have ingredients that are meant to provide the nails with a tough coating.

Nail strengtheners

These are usually clear and have nourishing and strengthening ingredients to help weak nails grow.

Cream nail varnish

Cream nail varnish is better for nails with many ridges and dents, as it does not show them up. The basic rule with cream nail varnish is:

- base coat
- two coats of cream varnish
- top coat.

Pearlised nail varnish

Pearlised nail varnish contains ingredients that give it a shimmery look. However, it shows up uneven surfaces in the nail plate, so should not be used on nails that are not healthy looking and smooth. With pearlised varnishes, the basic rule is:

- base coat
- two or three coats of varnish
- no top coat.

Solvents

Although not a varnish product, solvents are used to dissolve nail varnishes from furniture and clothes if they have been spilled, although this process is not always completely successful. However, the main use of solvent is to thin out nail varnishes when they become thick and sticky. A few drops in a bottle of varnish when shaken gives new life to a varnish, leaving it as thin as when it was first opened.

Top tip

Base coats and top coats can be used if a client wants a clear varnish instead of a colour varnish.

Get ahead

Investigate the ingredients found in nail varnishes and how the ingredients in different ones vary. For example, what ingredients are different in a pearlised nail varnish and a hardener? Make a poster or leaflet to show the ingredients in each product.

Carry out nail services (5)

The ingredients in nail varnish

It may help you to know more about the main ingredients in nail varnish and what they do. This information is presented in the table below.

Ingredient	Purpose
Nitrocellulose and resin	Carry the colour
Ethyl acetate	Helps speed up the drying time
Plasticiser	Makes the varnish flexible
Pigments	Gives colour
Bentonite clay	Stops colour separating

Choosing a nail varnish colour

Nail varnish comes in many colours. As a beauty therapist, you need to be aware of a few things before you can help your client choose the best nail varnish colour.

The length of the nails

Very bright colours on short or bitten nails will only draw attention to them and make the nails look shorter than they are.

The condition of the cuticles

Red-looking **cuticles** can look worse if the nails are painted in a bright or pearlised varnish. Pale and neutral colours in a cream varnish look better.

The client's home life and job

If a client has a job that could cause the nails to chip quite quickly, it is best to have a colour that is not going to show the odd little chip too much.

The client's skin colour

Orange, peach or beige colours show up the bluish colour in skin with poor circulation. Pinks clash with reddish skin tones.

The condition and smoothness of the nails

Pearlised varnish will show up any imperfections such as dents and ridges, so use a ridge-filling base coat and a cream varnish.

The size of the fingernails

Dark colours make the nails look smaller.

Get up and go!

Make a nail varnish chart that can be showed to the client. Get a piece of white card and place blobs of different coloured nail varnish on it. This will take a while to dry, perhaps even overnight. When the blobs are dry, label them all with the names of the varnishes. Keep this card in your portfolio and when doing your nail treatments allow the client to choose from the colours at the start.

Specialised treatments

Basic manicures and pedicures can be added to so that they become specialised. Here are some examples:

- exfoliating treatments – a rough cream is massaged into the feet and ball of the foot in circular movements to remove dead dry skin. It also improves the circulation and appearance of the skin
- foot or hand treatment mask – this can be applied at different stages of the treatment depending on the requirements. The hands or feet are then put into thermal booties to help the mask work better. The treatment improves the circulation, removes dead skin cells and softens the skin
- paraffin wax – a heated wax is applied to the hands or feet with a brush. The effects stimulate the circulation, help aches and pains and soften the skin.

Salon life

Penny had done a brilliant job of a manicure on Mrs Aziz but realised that she had not asked her client to choose a varnish colour at the start. Penny got the box of varnish colours and asked her client to choose a colour. Mrs Aziz chose the midnight black but, unfortunately, when Penny tried to open it, it was stuck.

Penny ran it under warm water and eventually managed to open the bottle top. The trouble was it was sticky and thick, and Penny knew that it would not go on very well, so she poured in some nail varnish remover and it thinned out really well.

Penny started to paint the fingernails but halfway through the varnish started to thicken again and it went on in a very lumpy and uneven way which made Mrs Aziz complain.

Is nail varnish remover a good way to thin a nail varnish? If not, what would be the best way to do this?

Why did the varnish start to thicken again?

Was the salon to blame in any way?

Carry out nail services (6)

Step-by-step manicure

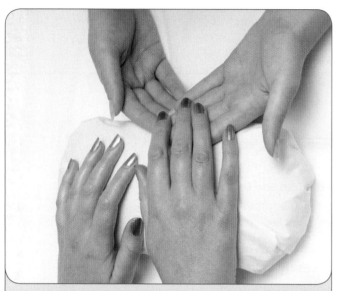

1   Wipe over the front and back of your client's hands with antiseptic. Carry out a consultation and check for contra-indications. Protect your client's sleeves with tissue.

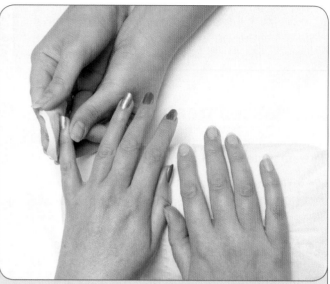

2   Left hand. Soak a clean ball of cotton wool with nail varnish remover. Hold on to the **nail plate** briefly, then wipe downwards to remove the dissolved varnish. Cover an orange stick with cotton wool, dip the end in nail varnish remover, and use this to go around the cuticle and nail fold.

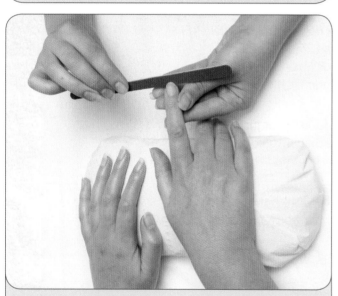

3   Right hand. File the nails using the fine side of the emery board.

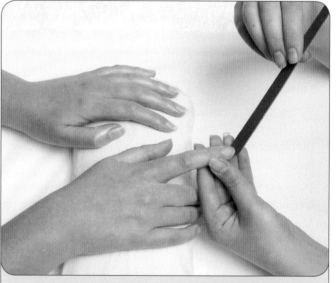

4   Right hand. Turn the emery board lengthways to the nail and very gently buff the tip of the nail with the fine side. This action is called bevelling. Bevelling seals the free edges of the nail, which prevents them from splitting and peeling back.

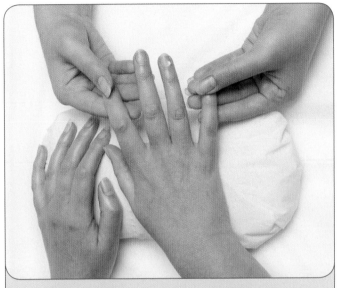

5 Right hand. Use a clean spatula to scoop out a small amount of cuticle cream. Dip a covered orange stick into the cream and apply it to the centre of the cuticles on each nail. Massage in the cuticle cream in a circular action so that it covers the nails and cuticles.

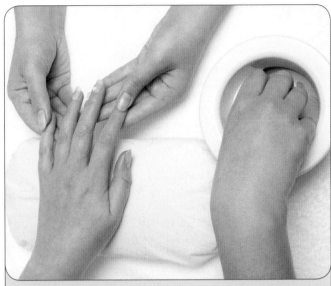

6 Place your client's right hand in a bowl containing warm soapy water. Repeat steps 2–6 on the client's left hand.

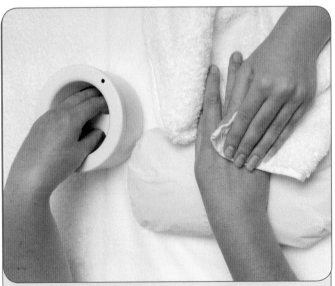

7 Take your client's right hand out of the water. Place the client's left hand in the water.

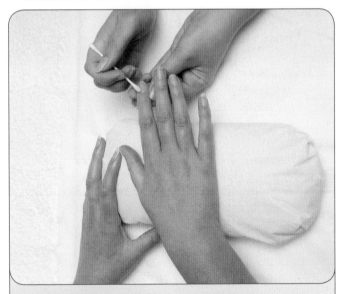

8 Dry your client's hand thoroughly, pushing the cuticles back with the towel. The senior therapist will then use a clean covered orange stick or cotton bud to apply cuticle remover to the cuticles and underneath the free edge. They will push back gently using circular actions, and clean under the free edge.

Carry out nail services (7)

Step-by-step manicure

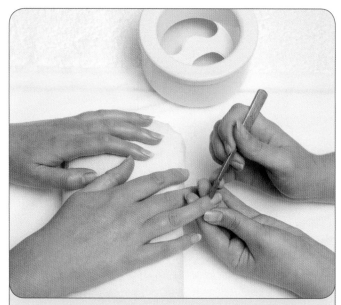

9   The senior therapist may need to ease away any excess cuticle with a cuticle knife. If there are any **hangnails** or loose bits of skin on the cuticles, she will also need to use the cuticle nippers to remove them.

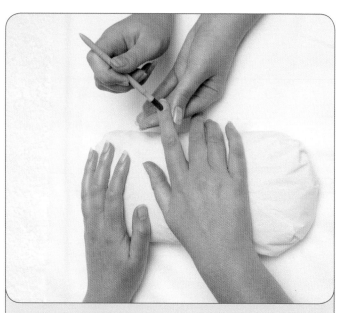

10   Remove the last traces of cuticle remover with a damp piece of cotton wool. Finally push back the treated cuticle with a rubber hoof stick.

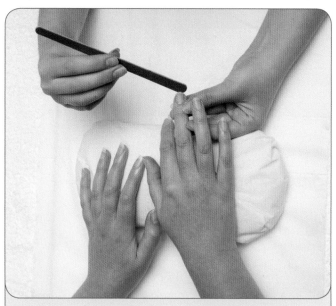

11   Take the client's right hand out of the water. Repeat steps 8–10 on the client's left hand. Tidy up the free edges of the nails on both hands with the emery board because very fine wisps of nail may have appeared, called **scarf nail**.

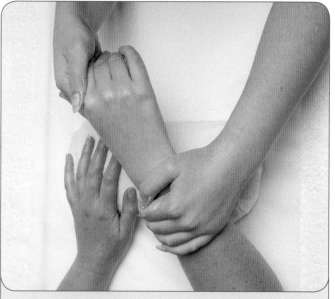

12   Using a spatula, place a small amount of massage cream or hand cream into the palm of your hands. Stroke the cream on to the skin of your client's arms using smooth upward effleurage movements.

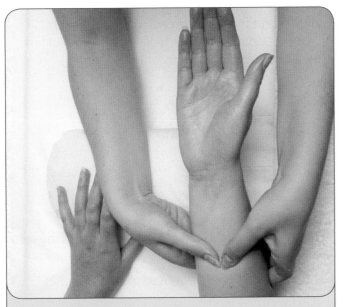

13 Massage using a variety of flowing effleurage and gentle kneading (petrissage) movements.

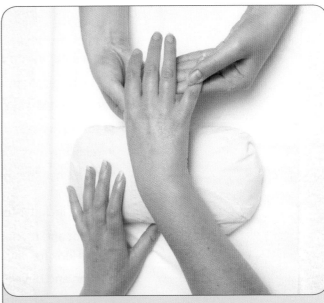

14 Finally, use petrissage techniques on the backs of both hands. Hand massage should take about five minutes.

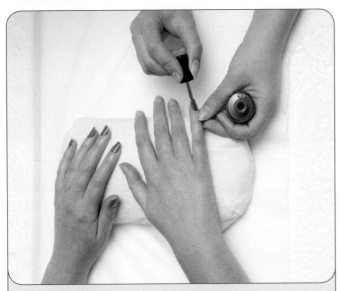

15 If you are going to buff your client's nails, do so at this point. Otherwise proceed with painting your client's nails. Go over the nail with nail varnish remover to degrease the **nail plate**, as you did at the start of your manicure. Paint the nails, following the routine described on pages 301 to 302.

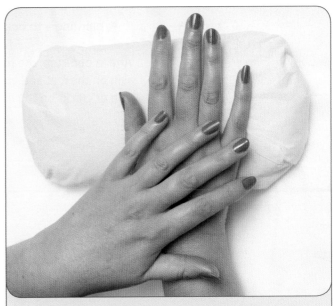

16 Check the finished result – the paint or polish completes the look.

Carry out nail services (8)

Pedicures

Pedicures are similar to manicures except that they are carried out on the feet instead of the hands. They improve the condition of the feet and toenails and take about an hour to complete. The aims of a pedicure are to:

- clean and shape the nails
- care for the cuticles
- soften dry skin on the feet, especially the heels
- relax the muscles in the leg and foot
- give a healthy shine to the nails.

A pedicure includes the following:

- a foot and toenail inspection – to check the condition of the skin on the feet and look for any problem areas
- filing and bevelling – to neaten the nails and remove splits and catches
- soaking – to soften the skin for cuticle work
- cuticle work – to push back and neaten the cuticles
- hard skin removal – using a foot file, rasp or **pumice stone**
- massage – to moisturise the skin, improve blood flow and relax the client
- **buffing** – to smooth ridges, give a healthy shine and improve the blood flow
- painting – to beautify the nails by adding colour and shine.

After a pedicure, the nails should look naturally polished or perfectly painted. The skin on the feet and around the cuticles should be soft and smooth without any hard skin or cracks on the heels.

Step-by-step pedicure

Start

1 Preparation and consultation

2 Check for contra-indications

3 Remove varnish

4 File and bevel

5 Cuticle massage cream

6 Soak

7 Cut toenails if necessary

8 Cuticle work

9 Rough skin remover

10 Massage and moisturise

11 Painting or buffing

Finish

Summary of steps in a pedicure

> **? Memory jogger**
>
> 1 List three nail-painting tips.
> 2 What is the purpose of buffing?
> 3 Why should you wipe over the nails with nail varnish remover before painting them?
> 4 What is a solvent?
> 5 What type of nail varnish is better for nails with ridges and dents?

Carry out nail services (9)

Step-by-step pedicure

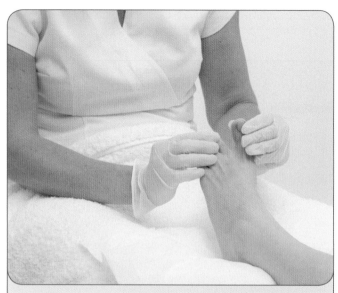

1   Wipe over the front and back of your client's feet with antiseptic. Carry out a consultation and check for contra-indications. Protect your client's trousers or skirt with a towel and couch roll for protection against water splashes and creams and lotions.

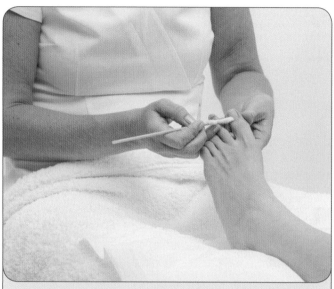

2   First foot. Soak a clean ball of cotton wool with nail varnish remover. Hold onto the **nail plate** briefly, then wipe downwards to remove the dissolved varnish. Cover an orange stick with cotton wool, dip the end into some nail varnish remover, and use this to go around the **cuticle** and nail fold.

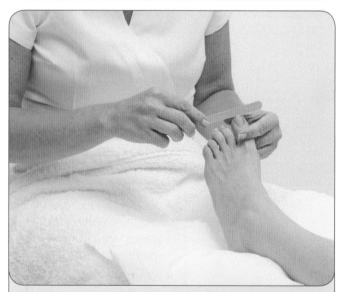

3   If the toenails don't need cutting (the senior therapist will cut them after they have been soaked), file the nails on the first foot using the coarse side of the emery board, unless the toenails are thin, in which case you will need to use the fine side.

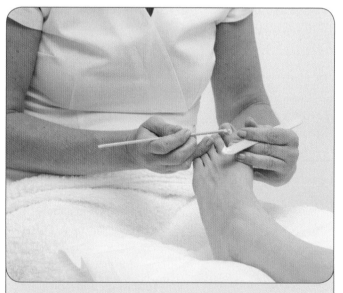

4   First foot. Turn the emery board lengthways and very gently buff the tip of the nail with the fine side. Use a clean spatula to scoop out some cuticle cream. Dip a covered orange stick into the cream and apply it to the centre of the cuticles on each nail. Massage in the cream in a circular action.

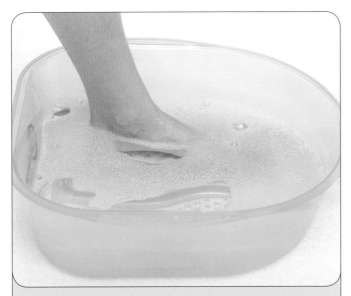

5   Place your client's first foot in the bowl or foot spa containing warm soapy water. On the client's second foot, repeat steps 2– 4.

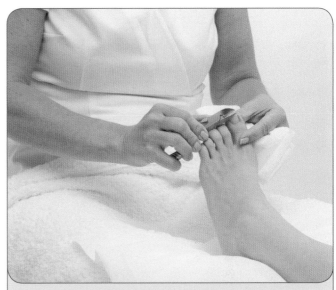

6   Take the client's first foot out of the water. Place the client's second foot in the water. Dry the client's first foot and nails thoroughly using a towel, pushing back the cuticles with the towel as you go. The senior therapist may now cut the toenails if necessary.

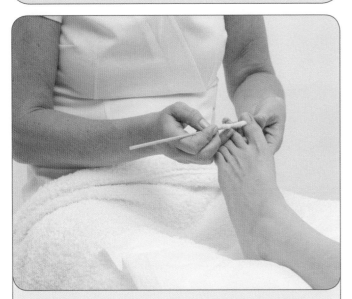

7   On the first foot, the senior therapist will use a clean covered orange stick to apply cuticle remover to the cuticles of each nail and underneath the free edge. When she has finished, take the orange stick, push back gently using circular actions, and clean under the free edge.

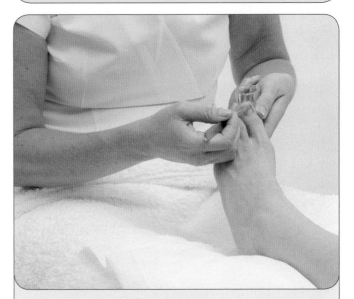

8   The senior therapist may need to ease away any excess cuticle with a cuticle knife. If there are any **hangnails** or loose bits of skin on the cuticles she will also need to use the cuticle nippers to remove them.

Carry out nail services (10)

Step-by-step pedicure

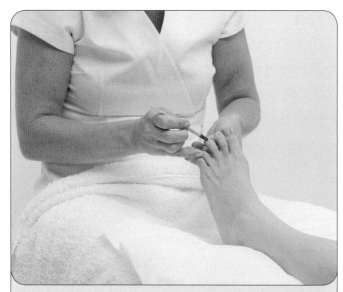

9 Remove the last traces of **cuticle** remover with damp cotton wool. Throw it away. Push back the treated cuticle with a rubber hoof stick. Take the client's other foot out of the water. Dry the foot and nails thoroughly, pushing back the cuticles with the towel. Repeat steps 7–9 on this foot.

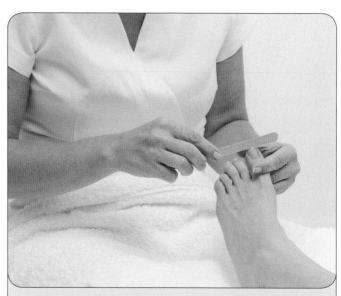

10 Tidy up the free edges of the nails on both feet with the emery board because very fine wisps of nail may have appeared, called **scarf nail**.

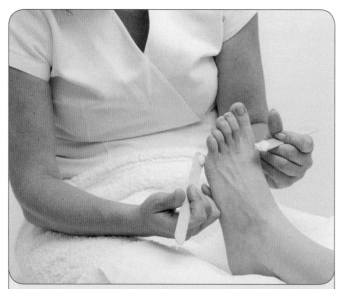

11 You may apply rough skin remover to the areas that need attention, most commonly the ball of the foot, the heel and side of the big toe. The senior therapist can use a foot rasp here if the skin is very rough.

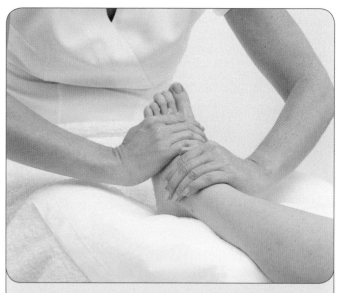

12 Using a spatula, place a small amount of massage cream into the palm of your hands. Stroke the cream on to the skin of your client's feet and legs using smooth upward effleurage movements. The muscles in the lower leg are quite strong and a deep massage will help to relax them.

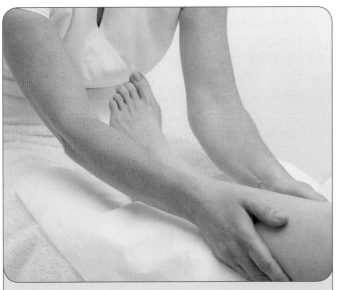

13 Massage using a variety of flowing effleurage and gentle kneading (petrissage) movements.

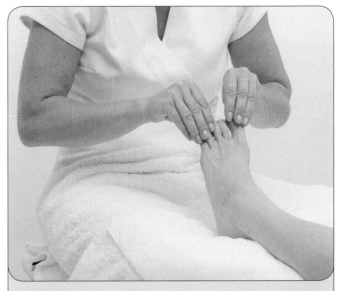

14 Finally, use petrissage techniques on the toes of both feet. Foot and leg massage should take about five minutes.

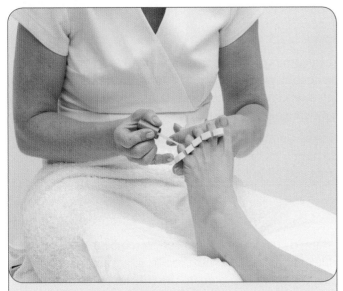

15 If you are going to buff your client's nails, do so at this point. Otherwise proceed with painting your client's nails. Go over the nail with nail varnish remover to degrease the **nail plate**. Paint the nails, following the routine described on pages 301 to 302.

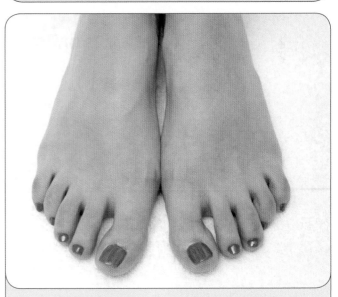

16 Check the finished result – the paint or polish completes the look.

Provide aftercare advice

Checking client satisfaction

When the whole manicure or pedicure and painting treatment is complete, you will need to check that the client is happy with the result. The easiest and most obvious way is to ask her. If there is anything that she is not happy about, then it is your job to put it right with the help of your supervisor.

If the client is satisfied with her treatment, you will then need to check that the finished effect meets the senior therapist's approval and that you completed the treatment within a commercially viable time (see page 320–321).

Next, you will need to complete the record card, adding anything about the treatment and products used as well as any information about how the treatment went.

 Top tips

- Leaving your work area clean and tidy ready for the next treatment is essential. Replace all furniture, put away products, replace dirty laundry, wipe surfaces, re-sterilise tools and get clean disinfectant.
- If the client is happy with her manicure and likes the products that you have used, it would be a good idea to ask her if she would like to look at the products on sale. Handy take-home packs are a good selling point, as they allow the client to continue with her nail care at home.

Male nails

Salon treatments for men are becoming more popular. Manicures and pedicures are especially popular as men like to look well groomed. The basic routine is the same – the only difference is that men tend to have their nails buffed instead of painted. Some men, however, do like a clear coat of varnish to give their nails a healthy shine.

Men who do manual jobs, such as car mechanics and builders, may have untidy and tough **cuticles**. They may also have a lot of staining to the nails, cuticles and under the free edge, so make sure that you have a very good cuticle remover.

 Top tip

For men with tough and stained cuticles, apply the cuticle remover generously, then leave it on for a couple of minutes. This will give the active ingredient sufficient time to bleach out the stains and prepare the cuticles for further treatment.

Homecare advice

After the manicure or pedicure, you should advise your client on how best to look after her nails so that they remain in the best condition.

The following list is good homecare advice for clients.

1   Wear rubber gloves when washing up or using strong cleaning products.

2   Keep hand cream by the sink and apply it after washing up. Wear hand cream at night.

3   Wear gardening gloves – don't use bare hands in the garden.

4   Don't use your nails as tools as this will weaken or break them.

5   Rinse off harsh products from the skin immediately as they could cause a rash or soreness.

6   Remove rings before washing so that soap does not build up under the rings and irritate the skin.

7   If there is a split on the nail, bevel it gently as soon as possible. (You may have to show your client what to do.)

8   Keep an emery board with you at all times so that you can smooth away any catch in the nail instantly.

9   Apply a top coat of polish over painted nails every other day, to make the varnish last longer.

10 Don't be tempted to pick dry **cuticles** – use a rich cream to soften them.

11 Always use a base coat under varnish to protect the nails from becoming stained.

12 Try to make time for a manicure every two weeks.

13 Try to make time for a pedicure every month.

14 Change socks or tights daily.

15 Make sure that footwear fits properly and is not tight.

16 Always file nails straight across.

17 Avoid wearing high heels for long periods of time.

18 Apply moisturiser to the feet after showering and having a bath.

>> Get up and go!

Take photos of your own or your partner's hands and feet before and after a treatment. Use these to make a poster advertising the benefits of a manicure and pedicure. Remember to make it colourful and eye-catching.

? Memory jogger

1   List four pieces of aftercare advice you could give to a client after a manicure.

2   List four pieces of aftercare advice you could give to a client after a pedicure.

Getting ready for assessment

Evidence requirements

You will be observed by your assessor on at least three occasions, one of which must be on the feet.

What you must cover during your practical assessments

Ranges

In your candidate handbook you will have a list of ranges that you must cover during your assessment. These ranges cover:

1 consultation techniques

2 nail finish

3 advice.

From the range you must show that you:

- have used all consultation techniques
- have applied three of the four types of nail finishes
- have provided all advice.

It is good practice to cover as many ranges as possible during each assessment. This will prevent you having to take too many additional assessments because there are many ranges that you have not managed to cover.

Performance criteria

What you must demonstrate during a practical observation by your tutor:

- preparation for nail treatments
- an assessment of the condition of skin and nails
- good communication skills
- basic nail care treatments
- checking the client is happy with the treatment and finished effect
- giving aftercare advice to the client
- leaving the work area in a suitable condition.

Throughout your observations you will also need to make sure that you pay attention to health, safety and hygiene throughout, as well as presenting yourself well, so read through Unit G20 Make sure your own actions reduce risks to health and safety before any practical assessment just to refresh your memory.

Carrying out a practical treatment using unhygienic tools, or without carrying out a risk assessment of your work area to avoid accidents happening, will mean that you are not safe to do a treatment and therefore could mean that you do not pass your assessment.

What you must know

In order to pass this unit, you will need to gather evidence during the teaching and learning of this unit before your assessor observes your practical performance. You will gather this during class work and further study and will probably file it in a portfolio of evidence. This evidence will also be signed off in your candidate handbook which you will be given by your assessor. This will be an official record to show that you have covered what you need to.

 Salon life

During a consultation with her client, Eve realised that what the client wanted was not in her best interests. The client's nails were dry and brittle, and the cuticles were very hard and slightly inflamed with skin that had grown along the nail plate. The client wanted a basic manicure and her nails painted a bright red colour – she had brought the colour in herself.

Very politely, Eve set about advising her client that, rather than a basic manicure, her nails needed some tender care.

What homecare advice should Eve provide to the client to get her nails back into good condition?

 Get up and go!

Investigate the products that you can buy to improve the condition of the nails at home. Create a poster with the pictures of the products and a brief description of what they do. Visit www.pearsonhotlinks.co.uk and search for this title for links to websites that will help you with this.

Treatment times and prices

Cost effectiveness and commercial viability

The commercially acceptable treatment time is the time that you need to take to carry out a treatment, from the client consultation process through to the aftercare advice, while still making money for the salon.

If you take longer than the time that is commercially acceptable to complete a treatment during your assessment, you will not pass because you will not be competent.

If you took too long to complete all your treatments, you wouldn't be able to fit many treatments into one day. You would therefore fail to make much money for the business and this would be commercially unacceptable. When you are working in a salon you should keep to the correct times. If you don't, you will fit in fewer clients – for example, just three instead of six in one day. This will mean the salon will lose money and clients will be kept waiting. Not being commercially viable could mean that your manager decides that you need a course of re-training to bring your skills up to speed and the worst case scenario if you still didn't improve is that you could lose your job. So you can see how important completing the job in the correct time is!

Although it is better for a client not to be rushed out after her treatment, it is not a good idea to leave the client too long in the treatment room once the treatment has finished. This would mean that the treatment room is not available for the next client, and that the therapist is late in starting her next treatment. This delay could then have a knock-on effect for the rest of the day. By the time the last client is seen, the therapist could be an hour or so behind schedule.

To avoid the treatment room being held up in this way, the best solution is to have a relaxing area where a client can sit quietly and have a drink after her treatment. Alternatively, if the salon is large and has many treatment rooms, then it is possible that the next treatment could start in a different room while the client is left to relax where she is.

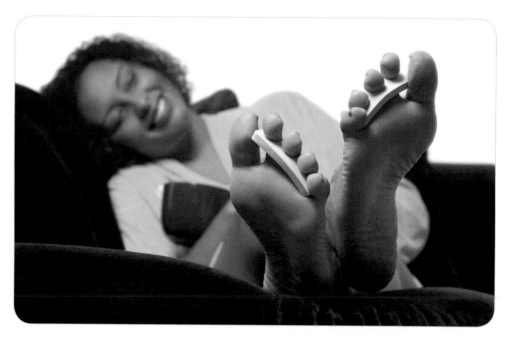

Recommended treatment times for Level 1 Certificate (NVQ/SVQ) in Beauty therapy

Service (excluding consultation and preparation)	Max time (mins)	Previous time (mins)
Assist with facial skin care treatments	30	45
Assist with nail services	30	30
Apply day make-up	30	New

Salon pricing

Pricing for beauty treatments and services varies from UK regions and town and city areas. Depending on the popularity of the area or type of salon, prices may be up to double the amount of that in another place. So it is difficult to state how much a client would expect to pay for a treatment.

≫ Get up and go!

1 Choose six towns in the UK.
2 Research the salons offering make-up treatments in the six towns by using a search engine and typing in 'beauty salons in <name of the place>'.
3 When you have your search results click on one of the salons, and see if they have a downloadable brochure which gives the list of treatments they offer and the prices. If not they may just list their prices on their website.
4 Do this until you have six prices for a treatment of your choice.
5 Print off the brochures and highlight the treatments.

⬆ Get ahead

- Create a graph to show the range of prices.
- Compare the prices and show the results to your class group. Discuss your findings.

Index